The Dementia Mastery Bible: Your Blueprint For Complete Dementia Management

Dr. Ankita Kashyap and Prof. Krishna N. Sharma

Published by Virtued Press, 2023.

THE DEMENTIA MASTERY BIBLE: YOUR BLUEPRINT FOR COMPLETE DEMENTIA MANAGEMENT

First edition. November 13, 2023.

Copyright © 2023 Dr. Ankita Kashyap and Prof. Krishna N. Sharma.

ISBN: 979-8223045595

Written by Dr. Ankita Kashyap and Prof. Krishna N. Sharma.

Table of Contents

DISCLAIMER

The information provided in this book is intended for general informational purposes only. The content is not meant to substitute professional medical advice, diagnosis, or treatment. Always consult with a qualified healthcare provider before making any changes to your diabetes management plan or healthcare regimen.

While every effort has been made to ensure the accuracy and completeness of the information presented, the author and publisher do not assume any responsibility for errors, omissions, or potential misinterpretations of the content. Individual responses to diabetes management strategies may vary, and what works for one person might not be suitable for another.

The book does not endorse any specific medical treatments, products, or services. Readers are encouraged to seek guidance from their healthcare providers to determine the most appropriate approaches for their unique medical conditions and needs.

Any external links or resources provided in the book are for convenience and informational purposes only. The author and publisher do not have control over the content or availability of these external sources and do not endorse or guarantee the accuracy of such information.

Readers are advised to exercise caution and use their judgment when applying the information provided in this book to their own situations. The author and publisher disclaim any liability for any direct, indirect, consequential, or other damages arising from the use of this book and its content.

By reading and using this book, readers acknowledge and accept the limitations and inherent risks associated with implementing the strategies, recommendations, and information contained herein. It is always recommended to consult a qualified healthcare professional for personalized medical advice and care.

Introduction

When you look in the mirror, have you ever wondered who is looking back at you? Not in the typical reflective sense, mind you, but with a tinge of confusion over the complex web that time has woven over your features. There's no denying that as we age, but what happens when our minds start to fail us? When the stories, the memories, and the treasured times vanish into thin air like whispers?

The word "dementia," which connotes uncertainty and fear, has invaded the lives of countless people. But do not worry, dear reader; the secret to solving the puzzles of dementia care is contained inside the pages of this little but powerful book. Welcome to my world, where I have explored the many facets of scientific study and medical journals, delving deeply into the maze-like tunnels of knowledge in an attempt to discover the mysteries of this puzzling ailment.

I'm Dr. Ankita Kashyap, a holistic healthcare and wellness advocate, a body and soul healer, and your mentor as you navigate the world of dementia mastery. It became obvious to me as I took up the gauntlet to write this ground-breaking work that I needed to create a healthy balance between medical knowledge and the subtle touch of holistic health. For this reason, I have combined the knowledge of credible scientific sources with the insight of other viewpoints to create a painstakingly arranged tapestry.

But enough about me; let's start this adventure together, my reader. I'll be your compass here in the Dementia Mastery Bible, guiding you toward the shores of empowerment, empathy, and understanding. Every page has been created with one goal in mind: to deliver you insightful knowledge and useful tactics that specifically address your difficulties.

The days of confusing medical jargon that made us feel even more lost than when we started are long gone. No, my dear reader, simplicity is king in this domain. I've made a deliberate decision to use simple language—a symphony of words meant to calm rather than confuse. We cannot navigate the maze of dementia unless we have clarity and insight.

Envision, if you will, a world in which relevance and adaptability serve as pillars for your journey and where information truly is power. Inside the sacred corridors of this literary haven, I provide you with individualised programmes and self-help methods that are meticulously crafted to suit the specific circumstances of your case. You are a treasured part of life's magnificent symphony, not just a name on a page.

As a healer, it is my responsibility to embrace the complex needs of my patients in addition to educating them. Because dementia affects everyone, it affects our friends, family, and communities. It is a menacing shadow that threatens to rob us of our most treasured memories. But do not be alarmed; together, we will dispel this darkness and arm ourselves with the information and resources needed to take it on head-on.

We will examine the various aspects of dementia mastery in the upcoming chapters. Our pursuit of empowerment and understanding will not stop at medical management or holistic approaches. I will impart to you the most recent findings, insights supported by data, and ageless knowledge that is just waiting to be found.

So, dear reader, if you have ever faced uncertainty or the hopelessness that comes with dementia, please take my hand and go with me into the realm of possibilities. Let's put the fear behind us and seize the power at our disposal. By working together, we will be able to uncover the mysteries of the mind and create a tapestry of unbridled hope, compassion, and resilience.

Greetings and welcome to the Dementia Mastery Bible, which is your comprehensive guide to dementia care. Together with the sure hand of science, the soft touch of holistic treatment, and the unshakable spirit of exploration, let's set out on this amazing voyage.

Chapter 1: Understanding Dementia

What Is Dementia?

What really is dementia then? To put it simply, it's a syndrome marked by a severe enough deterioration in cognitive ability to cause problems with day-to-day functioning. But there are a lot of intricate details hidden in this seemingly simple statement that you really need to grasp. Though it frequently becomes more common as we age, dementia is not only a natural component of becoming older. It is a unique disorder, the extent of which can only be fully understood by delving deeply into the inner workings of the brain.

We must first distinguish dementia from the typical ageing process in order to start comprehending it. It is normal for our cognitive capacities to deteriorate somewhat as we become older. We might have trouble remembering things, have trouble multitasking, or notice a little slowdown in our processing speed. These alterations are typically not a reason for alarm as they are a typical aspect of ageing. But if these cognitive deteriorations worsen to the point where they materially affect our daily life, that might be a sign of dementia.

There are numerous varieties of dementia, each with unique traits and underlying reasons. About 60–80% of instances of dementia are caused by Alzheimer's disease, making it the most prevalent type of dementia. It is a neurodegenerative condition that worsens over time and impairs thinking, behaviour, and memory. Other forms of dementia include frontotemporal dementia, which is caused by the degeneration of the brain's frontal and temporal lobes, Lewy body dementia, which is characterised by aberrant protein deposits, and vascular dementia, which is brought on by reduced blood flow to the brain.

Dementia, in any form, stems from fundamental brain alterations that gradually transpire. These alterations can be seen using a variety of imaging methods, including PET or MRI scans, and they offer important new information about the processes underlying dementia development. The buildup of aberrant protein deposits in the brain is one of the main indicators of dementia. For instance, these deposits manifest as tau tangles and beta-amyloid plaques in Alzheimer's disease, which impair neurons' regular activity and ultimately cause them to die.

Dementia patients also have notable modifications to their brain's structure and function in addition to these protein abnormalities. The hippocampus, which is in charge of memory and learning, and the frontal lobes, which are engaged in executive functions like problem-solving and decision-making, are two areas of the brain where these alterations can be observed. The symptoms worsen and the person's capacity for independent functioning declines as dementia gradually affects various brain regions.

Dementia is caused by a variety of intricate and intricate processes. Even though the precise aetiology of the majority of dementia types is still unknown, scientists have made great strides toward figuring out the complex chain of events that triggers the disease's onset. Genetic factors are important; specific gene mutations raise the likelihood of dementia development. The illness may also arise as a result of environmental factors such head trauma and exposure to chemicals.

Comprehending the fundamental processes and alterations in the brain linked to dementia is essential for multiple purposes. First of all, it helps us identify and distinguish between various forms of dementia more accurately, which can guide management and treatment plans. Secondly, because many of these brain alterations take place years before symptoms appear, it emphasises the significance of early detection and intervention. Lastly, it establishes the foundation for prospective future interventions and treatments meant to impede or stop the advancement of dementia.

To sum up, dementia is a complicated and intricate illness that extends beyond the typical cognitive ageing losses. It's a disorder that has a variety of forms, each having distinct traits and underlying reasons of their own. For dementia to be effectively managed and treated, it is necessary to comprehend the underlying mechanisms and changes in the brain that accompany the disease. Only by having a thorough grasp of this debilitating illness will we be able to start creating the tools and plans need to successfully navigate the difficult path ahead.

Types of Dementia

It is important to recognise the differences between the different types of dementia and their associated symptoms in order to comprehend dementia. This information directs the creation of individualised treatment strategies in addition to aiding in the identification of the underlying cause of cognitive decline. The four most prevalent forms of dementia—vascular dementia, frontotemporal dementia, Alzheimer's disease, and mixed dementia—will be discussed in this subchapter.

1. Alzheimer's Disease:

With Alzheimer's disease accounting for 60–80% of cases, it is the most common type of dementia. It is a neurological condition that worsens over time and mostly impacts thinking, behaviour, and memory. People may initially have modest amnesia, but as time passes, this forgetfulness gets worse and worse, eventually resulting in severe memory loss and difficulties going about daily tasks.

Other cognitive abilities including language, reasoning, and perception are also affected as the condition worsens. The buildup of neurofibrillary tangles and amyloid plaques in the brain is a hallmark of Alzheimer's disease. These aberrant protein clusters cause brain cells to deteriorate and ultimately die because they obstruct communication between them.

Alzheimer's disease patients may experience disorientation, anger, mood changes, and bewilderment. They could find it difficult to identify familiar faces and locations and find it tough to communicate clearly. Loss of appetite, sleep difficulties, and behavioural abnormalities are also frequent.

2. Vascular Dementia:

The second most prevalent type of dementia after Alzheimer's disease is vascular dementia. It happens when the blood arteries supplying the brain sustain injury, which lowers blood flow and oxygen delivery. Small vessel disease, high blood pressure, and stroke are some of the illnesses that might cause this.

Depending on where and how much brain damage has occurred, vascular dementia symptoms might change. They could involve memory issues as well as challenges with reasoning, problem-solving, and attention. Additionally, some people may develop personality changes, melancholy, and mood swings.

Vascular dementia frequently advances sequentially, with symptoms getting worse following a string of small or large strokes, in contrast to Alzheimer's disease, which has a steady reduction in function. Age, diabetes, high blood pressure, smoking, and a history of cardiovascular disease are risk factors for vascular dementia.

3. Frontotemporal Dementia:

A less prevalent but significant cause of dementia is frontotemporal dementia (FTD), especially in people under 65. Degeneration of the frontal and temporal lobes of the brain, which regulate behaviour, personality, and language, is its hallmark.

Depending on which specific brain regions are affected, frontotemporal dementia symptoms might differ greatly from one another. Changes in behaviour, including impulsivity, disinhibition, and apathy, are frequently the initial indications of the illness. People could behave in a socially incorrect way or do the same things over and over. There may also be language-related issues, such as speech and comprehension issues.

Unlike Alzheimer's disease, frontotemporal dementia preserves memory throughout the early stages of the illness. But as the illness worsens, people may have cognitive decline in addition to memory issues. Frontotemporal dementia is known to be significantly influenced by genetic abnormalities, and certain cases are familial.

4. Mixed Dementia:

As the name implies, mixed dementia is the simultaneous occurrence of two or more dementia types. Alzheimer's disease and vascular dementia are most frequently combined. Due to overlapping symptoms that make it challenging to differentiate between distinct types of dementia, mixed dementia presents special diagnostic and treatment issues.

Cognitive decline is exacerbated when Alzheimer's disease and vascular dementia pathology interact in the brain. The alterations associated with vascular disease, such as minor infarcts and white matter lesions, as well as those associated with Alzheimer's disease, such as amyloid plaques and neurofibrillary tangles, must be recognised and treated.

The degree of comorbid diseases and the main pathology can affect the symptoms of mixed dementia. Common symptoms include mood swings, memory issues, and issues with language and executive functioning. In order to effectively manage mixed dementia, it is usually necessary to treat both the underlying causes and specific symptoms.

Comprehending the various forms of dementia is essential for precise diagnosis and efficient handling. Every type exhibits distinct traits and symptoms, necessitating individualised approaches to care and therapy. Healthcare practitioners can establish individualised solutions that maximise an individual's overall well-being and quality of life by determining the underlying cause.

The next section of the book will cover the diagnosis process for dementia, including the several examinations, examinations, and imaging methods that are used to determine the precise kind of dementia that is being experienced and to assess cognitive performance. To improve treatment outcomes and slow the advancement of cognitive loss, keep in mind that early detection and intervention are essential.

Causes and Risk Factors

I've devoted my career as a medical doctor and health and wellness coach to assisting people in achieving holistic healthcare and wellness. We will examine the possible causes and risk factors for dementia in this chapter, including age, lifestyle variables, genetic predisposition, and underlying medical disorders. It is essential to comprehend these elements in order to recognise dementia early and prevent it from developing.

Genetic Predisposition

In certain instances, hereditary factors can be linked to dementia. Certain people may inherit genes that make them more prone to developing specific kinds of dementia, such Alzheimer's disease. Recent developments in the field of genetics and dementia have provided important new insights into the particular genes and genetic variants that may be linked to this crippling illness.

Scientists have found a number of genes that may affect a person's likelihood of acquiring dementia through intensive research. The apolipoprotein E (APOE) gene is one such gene. Research has indicated that an increased risk of Alzheimer's disease is associated with the APOE ε4 allele, a specific variation of the APOE gene. It's crucial to remember that carrying this gene does not ensure that dementia will develop. It merely makes everything more susceptible overall.

Finding a genetic predisposition to dementia can be discouraging, but it also gives people the ability to take preventative action to lower their risk and postpone the start of symptoms. People with genetic predispositions can take charge of their cognitive health by adopting a healthy lifestyle and adhering to preventative measures.

Age as a Risk Factor

The biggest contributing factor to dementia risk is age. As people age, they become more susceptible to dementia, an illness that is increasingly common in older populations and is a global health concern. Even while dementia is not an unavoidable side effect of ageing, it's vital to recognise that vulnerability increases with age.

The ageing process in and of itself can be harmful to the brain. Natural anatomical and functional changes occur in the brain with age, including the build-up of plaques and tangles, which are characteristic symptoms of Alzheimer's disease. Dementia may occur as a result of these age-related changes in addition to other lifestyle factors.

It is important to remember that preserving cognitive health does not rely on age. People of all ages can lower their risk of dementia or postpone the start of symptoms by implementing lifestyle changes and preventive techniques. Age-related cognitive decline can be mitigated in older adults by introducing a healthy lifestyle into their regular activities.

Lifestyle Factors

A person's lifestyle has a significant impact on how dementia develops and advances. Several research works have emphasised how specific lifestyle decisions affect cognitive performance. We can address these lifestyle variables and provide clients with the tools they need to make good changes by taking a holistic approach to dementia management.

Exercise is an important consideration. Regular exercise has been demonstrated to offer protection against dementia. Exercise enhances cardiovascular health and increases the release of a protein called brain-derived neurotrophic factor (BDNF), which helps neurons develop and survive.

Sustaining brain health also heavily depends on eating a balanced diet. A diet high in fruits, vegetables, whole grains, lean meats, and healthy fats, akin to the Mediterranean diet, may help lower the risk of dementia, according to research. Conversely, a diet heavy in processed foods, sugar, and saturated fats has been linked to a higher risk.

Furthermore, social and mental stimulation play a significant role in the prevention of dementia. Reading, solving puzzles, picking up a new skill, or doing other intellectually challenging activities can all assist to maintain the brain resilient and active. Keeping up social ties and taking part in fulfilling interactions are additional factors that support cognitive health.

Underlying Health Conditions

Dementia may arise as a result of a few underlying medical disorders. It has been demonstrated that diseases including diabetes, hypertension, and cardiovascular disease raise the chance of cognitive impairment. Over time, the brain's function may be compromised by certain disorders that alter blood flow to the brain.

It's also thought that dementia is influenced by inflammation. Chronic inflammation can harm brain cells and hasten cognitive loss, regardless of the cause—a medical disease that is present at the time or lifestyle choices. People can lower their risk of dementia and improve their general well-being by treating and managing these underlying medical disorders.

Early Detection and Prevention Strategies

Effective dementia management requires early detection. Early detection of the signs and symptoms allows people to get access to the right support resources and timely medical attention. Frequent cognitive screenings can assist in identifying any changes in cognition and offer a chance for early intervention.

Delaying the onset of dementia and lowering its risk both depend heavily on preventative measures. People can actively preserve their cognitive health by putting the lifestyle changes covered in this chapter into practise. These tactics, which range from maintaining a balanced diet and regular exercise to building social networks and taking care of underlying medical issues, serve as the foundation for holistic dementia care.

The possible causes and risk factors for dementia have been covered in this chapter, with a focus on the significance of early detection and preventative measures. Through comprehension of these variables and implementation of a comprehensive strategy for managing dementia, people can regain authority over their mental health and improve their general standard of living. By working together, we can enable people to face the difficulties posed by dementia with dignity, grace, and competence.

Signs and Symptoms

The most well-known sign of dementia is probably memory loss, but it's crucial to realise that this condition goes beyond simple forgetfulness from time to time. It is common and chronic for dementia-related memory loss to interfere with day-to-day activities and make it more difficult to recall people, locations, and events. It's critical to create routines, make use of visual aids like calendars and reminder notes, and keep an environment that is encouraging and empathetic for people who are experiencing memory loss.

Confusion is another common sign of dementia and can take many different forms. Dementia patients may find it difficult to follow discussions, become disoriented in familiar environments, or struggle to make decisions. An atmosphere that is predictable and structured can be quite beneficial in managing confusion. Reducing misunderstandings and aggravation can also be achieved by using clear communication and straightforward directions.

Dementia frequently causes problems with language and communication, making it difficult for patients to express themselves or comprehend others. Isolation and frustration may result from this. There are methods, nonetheless, that can aid in closing this gap. Enhancing communication efficacy can be achieved by using clear and short language, giving enough time for conversation, and making use of gestures or visual aids. Maintaining a sense of connection and promoting understanding also require empathy and patience.

Changes in behaviour and mood are common in dementia patients. This might include everything from anxiety and despair to agitation and impatience. Both the dementia patient and their carers may find these emotional shifts upsetting. Taking part in enjoyable activities, keeping a regular schedule, and creating a peaceful and encouraging environment can all aid in the regulation of emotions. Furthermore, it's critical to recognise and proactively address triggers that can result in behavioural changes.

Individuals suffering from dementia are also prone to sleep disruptions, which can lead to additional challenges for both the person with dementia and their caregiver. Improved sleep hygiene can be attained by establishing a regular bedtime, furnishing a cosy sleeping space, and using relaxing methods. Taking care of any underlying medical issues is also essential because some physical illnesses can aggravate sleep disorders.

Apart from these typical indications, dementia can also impair motor skills and coordination, making it challenging to perform daily tasks like eating, dressing, and maintaining personal cleanliness. When it comes to assisting people in retaining their independence and learning coping mechanisms to deal with these difficulties, occupational therapy can be quite helpful. It could also be essential to make adjustments to the living space and acquire assistive technology in order to guarantee mobility and safety.

As a medical expert, I think that changing one's lifestyle and practising self-care can effectively manage the symptoms of dementia. Participating in mentally challenging activities, eating a nutritious, well-balanced diet, and exercising frequently can all improve general wellbeing and possibly slow the onset of dementia. It may also be helpful to incorporate supplementary methods like music therapy, aromatherapy, and relaxation exercises to help with anxiety reduction and relaxation enhancement.

Last but not least, I am aware of how emotionally and physically taxing it can be to care for someone with dementia. In order to overcome any obstacles they may encounter, caregivers must build a network of resources and seek out help. Guidance and much-needed relief can be obtained through counselling, support groups, and respite care. Maintaining caregiver well-being also requires taking pauses, engaging in self-care, and having reasonable expectations for oneself.

In conclusion, providing appropriate care and support for those with dementia necessitates an understanding of the ability to recognise the signs and symptoms of the condition. Caregivers and medical professionals can improve the quality of life for dementia patients by using practical strategies if they are aware of the common symptoms, which include memory loss, confusion, language and communication difficulties, mood and behaviour changes, sleep disturbances, challenges with coordination and motor skills, and difficulties with mood. My goal is that this subchapter will be an invaluable resource for comprehending and coping with these symptoms, enabling both dementia patients and their carers to move closer to the ideal level of dementia care.

Impact on Daily Life

An people suffering from dementia may find it exceedingly difficult to perform daily activities that they used to perform with ease and regularity. As a physician and health and wellness coach, I have personally experienced the difficulties that people with dementia encounter and the toll that it has on their general quality of life. In this section, I'll examine the several ways that dementia impacts day-to-day functioning and offer doable strategies to deal with these challenges.

One area of daily living that people with dementia find more and more difficult is self-care. Even basic activities like washing, clothing, and grooming can become difficult and perplexing. People suffering from dementia frequently experience difficulties remembering basic personal hygiene practises or coordinating the motions required for self-care. This can be discouraging and distressing, which lowers one's sense of self-worth and general wellbeing.

To tackle these obstacles, it's critical to create a regimented and streamlined self-care practise. For people suffering from dementia, breaking down tasks into smaller, more manageable steps helps increase their sense of control and confidence. Giving people visual cues—like written instructions or illustrated guides—can also help them remember things and become more independent. Including a loved one or caregiver who can provide helpful nudges and support without taking over the activity entirely can also help preserve a sense of autonomy.

Dementia patients also find it more and more difficult to do household activities. As the illness worsens, the capacity to handle money, prepare meals, do laundry, and keep one's home tidy can progressively deteriorate. For those accustomed to caring for themselves and their houses, this loss of independence can be upsetting and stressful.

It's critical to modify these activities to the capacities of people with dementia in order to preserve a sense of normalcy and avoid emotions of helplessness. The chores can be easier to manage if they are broken down into smaller phases and simplified. Another way to help with memory recall is to provide visual cues and reminders. For example, color-coding systems or labelling cabinets and drawers might make it easier for people with dementia to find things and get around.

To the best of their abilities, people with dementia must also be included in these tasks. This has advantages for their cognitive health in addition to preserving their feeling of value and purpose in life. Promoting involvement in domestic tasks can enhance mental abilities and offer a feeling of achievement. But it's crucial to recognise their limitations and offer assistance and direction only when necessary, without becoming overbearing.

Furthermore, because it fosters a sense of connection and belonging, maintaining social relationships is essential for those with dementia. However, social connections may become more difficult as the disease worsens and cognitive impairments worsen. Dementia patients may find it difficult to follow social cues, carry on conversations, or recall faces and names. They might withdraw and become solitary, which would make them feel depressed and alone.

It is crucial to create a compassionate and understanding atmosphere for people with dementia in order to support them in their social interactions. It is important to encourage friends, family, and caregivers to be understanding and patient. People with dementia can follow along and actively participate in conversations when they are simplified and language is used in a clear and concise manner. Participating in activities that emphasise reflection and past encounters is also advantageous because these might serve to evoke memories and create a feeling of familiarity.

Apart from these approaches, there exist other supplementary methods and coping strategies that persons suffering from dementia can integrate into their everyday routines to effectively handle the consequences on their general welfare. Regular physical activity can support the maintenance of both physical and mental health. Examples of this type of exercise are walking and moderate yoga. This can be further improved by including brain-stimulating activities in everyday routines, such as reading, playing music, or doing puzzles.

For those suffering from dementia, it's also critical to maintain a healthy, balanced diet. Studies have indicated that specific dietary adjustments, such adhering to a Mediterranean diet high in fruits, vegetables, whole grains, and lean proteins, can help prevent cognitive deterioration and enhance general brain function. Getting advice from a dietician or nutritionist can help people with dementia make wise decisions and make sure they are getting the nutrients they require.

Finally, self-care practises like mindfulness, deep breathing exercises, and relaxation methods can help people with dementia feel at ease and support their mental health. Encouraging artistic and self-expressional pursuits like writing, painting, or listening to music can also help them feel more like themselves and serve as a therapeutic release.

In summary, dementia has a substantial influence on day-to-day functioning and can negatively impair a person's independence and quality of life. However, people with dementia can retain some degree of independence and carry on with their favourite hobbies by putting the solutions and adaptations covered in this subchapter into practise. It's important to keep in mind that each person with dementia is different, and what works for one might not work for another. In order to ensure that people with dementia continue to lead happy and meaningful lives, it is crucial to modify these tactics to meet their unique needs and skills.

Progression and Stages

A neurodegenerative condition called dementia damages the brain and impairs thinking, reasoning, and memory. Because of its progressive nature, the illness gets worse with time. When dementia first appears, people may have little memory loss and have trouble with cognitively demanding tasks. But when the illness worsens, these symptoms worsen and interfere with day-to-day activities.

There are various stages in the development of dementia, each with its own set of symptoms and difficulties. I will talk about the widely accepted Global Deterioration Scale (GDS), which breaks the disease down into seven stages, even though there are several staging schemes available.

People in stage 1, sometimes referred to as normal ageing or no cognitive decline, do not exhibit any dementia-related symptoms. At this point, people may have occasional slight forgetfulness, but they can usually continue with their regular activities and function on their own.

The symptoms of stage 2, often known as mild cognitive impairment, include mild memory loss, difficulty focusing, and trouble solving problems. People going through this phase could have trouble speaking or recalling previous events. Nonetheless, people may still handle their everyday responsibilities with minor assistance, and these challenges are frequently disregarded as normal indications of ageing.

Early-stage dementia, or mild dementia, first appears in stage 3. This is when the person's loved ones start to observe the cognitive impairment more clearly. It's possible for memory loss, disorientation, and difficulties with routine tasks to worsen. People could also struggle to follow conversations or find the appropriate words. Their mounting difficulties may cause them to become withdrawn from social interactions or exhibit indications of frustration.

Significant cognitive deterioration is visible when dementia advances to stage 4, or mild dementia. As memory loss worsens, people may find it difficult to perform daily duties like grooming and clothing. They might also experience disorientation and struggle to identify familiar individuals or locations. During this phase, behavioural disturbances like agitation and impatience may also surface.

People reach the severe dementia stage by stage 5. Severe memory loss may make an individual need assistance with all everyday activities. They could struggle to communicate and grow more reliant on others for personal care. Delusions and other behavioural abnormalities are also possible. At this point, it is essential to create a safe, nurturing environment to guarantee the person's comfort and well-being.

The first signs of late-stage dementia appear in stage 6. People might not be able to communicate or understand language at this time. They might have trouble swallowing, which could result in weight loss and other health issues. As incontinence increases in frequency, assistance with toileting becomes necessary. People may become more and more immobile, needing assistance with mobility aids or becoming bedridden. They might start acting more erratically, exhibiting greater hostility, anxiety, or roaming.

People finally reach the final stage of dementia at stage 7. They rely entirely on others to take care of all personal hygiene, food, and clothing needs. They might have trouble swallowing and be more prone to getting sick. People's physical capacities keep deteriorating, and they can end up bedridden. Palliative care takes centre stage at this point, with the goals of comfort and symptom relief.

It is crucial to remember that every person's dementia progresses differently. Each stage's length and intensity can differ based on a number of variables, including the kind of dementia, general health, and unique circumstances. Furthermore, different symptoms may be experienced by different people at different phases, which complicates and makes it difficult to forecast the course.

It is essential for caregivers, medical experts, and dementia patients themselves to understand the stages of the disease. It facilitates the process of organising suitable care and assistance, making knowledgeable decisions on treatment and lifestyle adjustments, and fostering compassion and understanding for individuals impacted by the illness.

In my business, I collaborate closely with patients and their families to create individualised care plans that take into account each patient's unique requirements and dementia stage. Working with professionals from a range of health and wellness domains, such as psychologists, dieticians, and therapists, is part of this. Our combined goal is to offer comprehensive care that includes not just medical interventions but also counselling, lifestyle changes, and self-help methods.

It can be difficult to navigate the progression of dementia, but with the correct information, resources, and support, people and their loved ones can manage the illness more skillfully. Through comprehension of the various phases of dementia and the corresponding alterations in cognition, behaviour, and function, we can offer care and assistance that enhances general health and quality of life all the way through the dementia journey.

Diagnosis and Evaluation

In my capacity as a physician and wellness and health coach, I have had the honour of assisting people with a range of medical issues. Dementia, on the other hand, is a disorder that has long fascinated me. This degenerative illness affects the patient directly as well as posing special difficulties for family members and caregivers.

We examine the dementia diagnostic procedure in this subsection. I truly think that the key to effectively managing this issue is early diagnosis. Creating a thorough treatment plan requires an understanding of the imaging tests, medical examinations, cognitive testing, and diagnostic procedures.

The Diagnostic Process:

Accurate diagnosis is the first step towards managing and understanding dementia. A number of assessments and tests are used in the diagnostic procedure to identify the existence and degree of cognitive decline. It necessitates a comprehensive strategy combining medical experts from different fields.

1. Medical Evaluation:

A comprehensive medical evaluation is the first stage in the diagnosis process. A thorough medical history, including any family history of dementia or associated disorders, is required for this examination. Determining the probable reasons and contributing aspects of the patient's cognitive impairment requires assessing their medications, lifestyle choices, and previous and present symptoms.

2. Cognitive Assessment:

Evaluating cognitive function is crucial to dementia diagnosis. A variety of cognitive domains, including memory, attention, language, visuospatial skills, and executive function, are assessed in cognitive examinations. Healthcare practitioners can receive assistance in effectively assessing cognitive capacities from a number of approved instruments and tests, such as the Montreal Cognitive Assessment (MoCA) and the Mini Mental State Examination (MMSE).

3. Imaging Tests:

Imaging studies are essential to the diagnosis process because they reveal important details about the composition and operation of the brain. When examining the brain for any structural anomalies, such as shrinkage or the presence of plaques and tangles, which are frequently linked to various forms of dementia, magnetic resonance imaging, or MRI, is frequently utilised. Furthermore, variations in brain metabolism can be identified using Positron Emission Tomography (PET) scans that employ radioactive tracers, which helps distinguish between different forms of dementia.

Importance of Early Diagnosis:

Dementia patients and their carers stand to gain greatly from an early diagnosis. Proactive illness management is made feasible by timely intervention, giving patients the most quality of life possible. Furthermore, early diagnosis gives patients the ability to make plans for their future, including financial and legal ones, and to engage in decisions about their care.

1. Treatment Options:

An increasing array of dementia treatment options are now available due to advances in research and medicine. A timely diagnosis enables medical practitioners to start the right therapies as soon as possible, which may help to reduce the disease's course and relieve symptoms. In certain people, medications like memantine or cholinesterase inhibitors can improve and stabilise cognitive performance.

2. Lifestyle Modifications:

Lifestyle adjustments are essential for managing dementia in addition to medicine. When patients receive a diagnosis early, medical practitioners can help them and their carers make the appropriate lifestyle adjustments, including as eating a different diet, exercising frequently, engaging in cognitive stimulation, and learning stress-reduction strategies. Both general quality of life and cognitive function are maintained by these therapies.

3. Care Planning and Support:

Early diagnosis gives patients and their caregivers more time to make future plans and find the right kind of assistance. It makes it possible to locate neighbourhood resources, support networks, and caregiving services, ensuring that caregivers have the resources and help they need to successfully handle the difficulties brought on by dementia.

4. Research and Clinical Trials:

For those with dementia diagnoses, taking part in clinical trials or research studies is an additional alternative. Early diagnosis gives patients the chance to learn about ways they may progress medicine and even gain access to novel therapies or interventions. Dementia patients can actively contribute to the search for a treatment and the development of new management techniques by taking part in these research.

Conclusion:

A thorough assessment including medical exams, cognitive assessments, and imaging testing is necessary for the diagnosis of dementia. In order to enable patients and those who care for them to take proactive measures to manage the illness, obtain the right therapies, and make future plans, early diagnosis is essential. By employing a multidisciplinary strategy that includes medical interventions, lifestyle modifications, and support services, we can improve the general state of health and quality of life for all dementia patients.

Living With Dementia

Both the individual with dementia and their carers may find living with the disease to be an overwhelming experience. It necessitates a special strategy that takes into account each person's particular requirements and difficulties. I'll lay out a detailed plan in this chapter to assist you in adjusting to life with dementia gracefully and easily.

Creating a Safe and Supportive Environment

It's critical to create a secure and encouraging environment for those with dementia. This entails altering the physical area to discourage mishaps and encourage independence. These are some important things to remember:

1. Remove hazards: Evaluate the living area thoroughly and get rid of any possible threats. This could entail making sure that all paths are free, clearing clutter, and tying down any loose cords.

2. Enhance lighting: For those suffering from dementia, adequate lighting is crucial since it can increase safety and lessen confusion. Install non-glare, bright lighting throughout the house, with a focus on the bathrooms, stairwells, and hallways.

3. Install safety devices: To stop falls and accidents, think about adding safety features like grab bars, handrails, and nonslip mats. Additionally, think about utilising monitoring systems or sirens that can notify caretakers of crises.

4. Simplify the environment: Too many things or sensations can overwhelm a person suffering from dementia. Reduce visual clutter, use minimalist décor, and arrange items so they are easily accessible to simplify the space.

Managing Daily Routines

People with dementia may feel more safe and in control of their lives if they establish and adhere to a regimented daily schedule. Additionally, it can lessen disorientation and anxiety. Here are a few pointers for organising daily schedules:

1. Establish a daily schedule: Make a daily plan that incorporates necessary tasks like taking care of oneself, exercising, eating, and remembering to take medications. Show off the schedule in a way that is easy to see, like on a large calendar or whiteboard.

2. Foster independence: By dividing up work into manageable chunks and offering visual clues or suggestions, you can promote independence. To help remind the person to brush their teeth, you may, for instance, put a toothbrush and toothpaste next to the sink.

3. Allow flexibility: Allowing for flexibility and adaptability is crucial, even though structure is also necessary. Recognize that the individual's capabilities might shift over time, and be ready to adjust the routine appropriately.

4. Incorporate meaningful activities: Get the person involved in important and enjoyable activities. Hobbies, crafts, puzzles, and music listening may all fall under this category. Engaging in meaningful activities can enhance mood, mental clarity, and general wellbeing.

Accessing Community Resources

Being a person with dementia does not mean that you have to go alone. Making use of community services can help the person in need as well as their caretakers by offering important support and assistance. Here are some directions to investigate:

1. Support groups: Participating in a support group can be very helpful for both carers and those who are suffering from dementia. These groups offer a forum for exchanging experiences and coping mechanisms as well as a feeling of belonging and understanding.

2. Day care programs: Day care centres created especially for people with dementia can provide caregivers a break while giving the person with dementia a secure and stimulating atmosphere. These programmes frequently involve social interaction, activities, and supervision.

3. Memory clinics: Memory clinics specialize in diagnosing and managing various forms of dementia. They provide comprehensive assessments, treatment plans, medication management, and ongoing

support. Consultation with a memory clinic can help ensure that all aspects of care are being addressed.

4. Financial assistance programs: Living with dementia can place a significant financial burden on individuals and their families. It is important to explore financial assistance programs available through government agencies, non-profit organizations, or healthcare facilities.

By following these steps, you can lay a solid foundation for living with dementia and promote a better quality of life for both the individual and their caregivers. Remember, each person's experience with dementia is unique, so it's important to tailor these strategies to meet their specific needs and preferences. Seek guidance from healthcare professionals specializing in dementia care, as they can offer personalized advice and support throughout the journey. Living with dementia is undoubtedly challenging, but with the right approach, it is possible to find moments of joy, connection, and fulfillment.

Chapter 2: Medical Management of Dementia

Medications for Dementia

As a physician and health and wellness coach, patients and their families frequently come to me for advice regarding the many dementia drugs. It is crucial to remember that although these drugs can aid in the management of cognitive symptoms, the fundamental causes of dementia cannot be cured or reversed. Nonetheless, they can enhance a patient's quality of life and offer some respite.

Cholinesterase inhibitors are one type of drugs that is frequently prescribed to treat dementia. Acetylcholine is a neurotransmitter that these drugs function by raising its levels in the brain. Acetylcholine is known to be reduced in dementia patients and is important in memory, attention, and other cognitive processes.

Galantamine, rivastigmine, and donepezil are the cholinesterase inhibitors that are most frequently administered. These drugs come in a variety of forms and dosages, including liquids, tablets, and patches for oral use. They can be applied to many kinds of dementia, such as Lewy body dementia, vascular dementia, and Alzheimer's disease.

The specific method by which cholinesterase inhibitors work is by blocking the acetylcholinesterase enzyme, which in the brain hydrolyzes acetylcholine. These drugs efficiently raise acetylcholine levels by blocking this enzyme, which improves cognitive performance in dementia patients.

Studies have demonstrated that cholinesterase inhibitors can help certain people perform better cognitively and slow down the rate at which cognitive decline occurs. Though the evidence is not as strong, they might also be helpful in controlling behavioural symptoms including aggression and agitation.

Cholinesterase inhibitors do, however, have the potential to cause negative effects, just like any medicine. These may consist of vomiting, diarrhoea, appetite loss, and insomnia. If any of these adverse effects manifest, it's critical to notify the healthcare professional so that alternate medications or dose modifications can be considered.

Medatine is another drug that is frequently used to treat dementia. The way this drug functions is by preventing the activation of the neurotransmitter glutamate. Since glutamate plays a role in the communication between nerve cells, high glutamate levels have been linked to the deterioration and death of nerve cells in dementia patients.

Although it can potentially be used for other forms of dementia, memantine is mainly used to treat moderate-to-severe Alzheimer's disease. It is typically taken once day and is available as an oral tablet.

In order to prevent overstimulating nerve cells, memantine works by controlling the activity of glutamate receptors in the brain. In doing so, it enhances cognitive performance in dementia patients and helps shield brain cells from additional harm.

According to research, memantine can help people with moderate-to-severe Alzheimer's disease by improving their cognitive and functional outcomes and offering some respite. Additionally, it might be helpful in controlling neuropsychiatric symptoms like aggressiveness and agitation.

Similar to cholinesterase inhibitors, memantine may cause adverse reactions. Constipation, headaches, dizziness, and confusion are a few of these. Once more, if any of these adverse effects manifest, it's crucial to notify the healthcare professional as they can need additional evaluation and treatment.

For patients with moderate to severe dementia, doctors occasionally prescribe a combination of memantine plus cholinesterase inhibitors. With this combined therapy, cognitive symptoms can be more effectively managed by addressing both the overstimulation of glutamate receptors and the depletion of acetylcholine in the brain.

It's critical to understand that although drugs can be useful in controlling cognitive symptoms in dementia patients, they are not a panacea. They function best when combined with other non-pharmacological strategies such cognitive stimulation, psychosocial therapies, and lifestyle changes.

Because everyone responds differently to various medications, it is also critical to routinely evaluate the safety and efficacy of these treatments. Depending on the individual needs of the patient and how they respond to treatment, dosage modifications or changes in medications may be necessary.

In my capacity as a health and wellness coach, I stress the value of managing dementia holistically. Medication is only one piece of the puzzle; you also need to take into account other aspects including social interaction, stress management, sleep, exercise, and nutrition.

To sum up, medicine can be a useful tool in the treatment of dementia, especially when it comes to treating cognitive symptoms. Memantine and cholinesterase inhibitors are two often given drugs that have been demonstrated to help people with dementia by improving their cognitive performance and offering some respite. But it's crucial to be aware of any possible negative effects and to routinely evaluate how well they work and how tolerable they are. For complete dementia management, a multimodal strategy that incorporates non-pharmacological and pharmaceutical interventions is essential.

Non-Pharmacological Interventions

Millions of people worldwide are afflicted with dementia, a complicated and fatal illness. A reduction in cognitive function, memory loss, poor judgement, and behavioural and personality abnormalities are its hallmarks. Although there isn't a cure for dementia at this time, there are a number of therapeutic options that can assist those who have the illness live better lives.

Pharmacological therapies, such as taking medicine to control symptoms and slow down the disease's progression, are frequently used in traditional dementia treatment options. Although these drugs have some potential benefits, they frequently have negative side effects and might not be suitable for everyone. Non-pharmacological therapies can help in this situation.

Interventions that do not entail the administration of pharmaceuticals are referred to as non-pharmacological interventions. Through a variety of therapeutic exercises, they aim to improve mood, promote overall well-being, and improve cognitive performance. Depending on the needs and desires of the patient, these interventions may be utilised as stand-alone therapies or in conjunction with pharmaceutical treatments.

Cognitive stimulation treatment is a non-pharmacological strategy that is frequently utilised in the management of dementia (CST). The goal of CST, an organised, group-based therapy, is to engage and stimulate dementia patients in a range of activities that are intended to enhance cognitive function. Puzzles, word games, memory tests, and topical debates are a few examples of these activities.

Studies have demonstrated the substantial advantages that CST can provide for dementia patients. According to a research in the British Medical Journal, people who had CST had increases in their memory and attention span, among other cognitive functions. They also mentioned feeling happier and having better general wellbeing.

A different study that was published in the Journal of the American Medical Association discovered that CST helped people with mild to moderate dementia with their communication, quality of life, and cognitive function.

Reminiscence therapy is an additional non-pharmacological strategy for dementia. During this therapy, objects, photographs, and other sensory aides are used to help people with dementia remember and communicate experiences from the past. Reminiscence therapy helps people with dementia interact, communicate, and feel better overall by drawing on long-term memories.

Studies have indicated that recollection therapy can benefit those suffering from dementia. According to a research in the Journal of Clinical Nursing, people who received recollection therapy showed increases in their social interaction, mood, and cognitive abilities. They also mentioned feeling more like themselves, having higher self-esteem, and having a better quality of life overall.

Another non-pharmacological strategy that has demonstrated promise in the treatment of dementia is music therapy. Music can stimulate memories, create strong emotional reactions, and enhance cognitive performance due to its potent brain-based effects. Singing, playing instruments, and listening to music are examples of musical activities that can be used in music therapy to engage people with dementia and enhance their emotional wellbeing.

Studies have indicated the advantages of music therapy for those suffering from dementia. According to a study that was published in the Journal of the American Geriatrics Society, people with dementia who received music therapy reported improvements in their conduct, mood, and general quality of life. Another study that was published in the Journal of Alzheimer's Disease discovered that music therapy helped dementia patients connect with others more socially and with less agitation.

Apart from music therapy, recollection therapy, and cognitive stimulation therapy, there exist various more non-pharmacological interventions that may prove advantageous for patients suffering from dementia. These interventions include of yoga and mindfulness exercises, aromatherapy, pet therapy, and art therapy.

Using artistic mediums like painting, drawing, and sculpting, art therapy enables people with dementia to express themselves and participate in the creative process. According to research, art therapy can help people with dementia feel better emotionally, behave less agitatedly, and generally be more well-rounded.

Interactions with animals, such as dogs or cats, are part of pet therapy, often referred to as animal-assisted therapy, which aims to enhance social, emotional, and physical well-being. Studies have indicated the advantages of pet therapy for those suffering from dementia, such as decreased agitation, elevated mood, and enhanced social engagement.

Essential oils are used in aromatherapy to improve mood and encourage relaxation. It has been discovered that certain essential oils, such lavender and lemon balm, have uplifting and relaxing benefits on dementia sufferers. Fragrant goods, massage oils, and diffusers can all be utilised in aromatherapy.

People with dementia may also benefit from yoga and mindfulness exercises. In order to encourage relaxation, lower stress levels, and enhance general wellbeing, these activities incorporate breathing techniques, gentle movements, and meditation. Studies have indicated that the application of yoga and mindfulness techniques can improve the quality of life for dementia patients by lowering anxiety and sadness and improving cognitive performance.

The treatment of dementia can be approached holistically and person-centeredly with non-pharmacological therapies. Through a variety of therapeutic exercises, they aim to improve mood, promote overall well-being, and improve cognitive performance. In addition to pharmacological therapies, these interventions can be customised to match the specific needs and preferences of people with dementia, enabling comprehensive dementia care.

In my experience as a physician and health and wellness coach, non-pharmacological approaches have been shown to be quite effective for people with dementia. I have personally seen the beneficial effects that these interventions can have on the lives of those who are dealing with this illness. Individuals with dementia may benefit from enhancements in their general well-being, mood, and cognitive function through the use of non-pharmacological therapies such as music therapy, recollection therapy, and cognitive stimulation therapy in their care plans. Despite the difficulties associated with dementia, these interventions provide individuals and their loved ones with hope and support, enabling them to have happy and meaningful lives.

Lifestyle Modifications

Regular exercise is one of the most important lifestyle changes I advise all of my patients to make. Exercise has been demonstrated to promote the release of endorphins, which are organic mood enhancers, as well as to assist maintain a healthy weight and cardiovascular health. It has been discovered that physical activity elevates brain-derived neurotrophic factor (BDNF), a protein that supports the development and endurance of nerve cells within the brain.

Exercise may seem difficult to include into a dementia patient's daily routine, but it is definitely not impossible. Even seemingly simple pursuits like dancing, walking, or gardening can have enormous benefits. It's crucial to select pursuits that the person finds enjoyable and safe to engage in. It is advised to work out under the guidance of a qualified professional, such as a physical therapist or licenced fitness teacher, to ensure safety.

Keeping up a healthy diet is another essential component of changing one's lifestyle to manage dementia. Studies have demonstrated the beneficial effects of a diet high in fruits, vegetables, whole grains, lean meats, and healthy fats on cognitive performance. These meals offer vital nutrients that promote mental wellness and guard against cognitive loss brought on by ageing.

A person with dementia has unique demands and restrictions that should be taken into account when designing a diet. For people who have trouble chewing or swallowing, this may entail changing the texture of the food. A healthy weight must be maintained, thus it's also critical to make sure the person is eating enough calories. It could be suggested to use dietary supplements in specific situations to meet nutritional needs.

Getting enough sleep is another essential dementia control strategy. Individuals suffering from dementia frequently experience sleep problems, which can significantly affect their cognitive abilities and general well-being. A regular sleep schedule and a conducive environment can both significantly enhance the quality of sleep.

Establishing a regular bedtime and wake-up time, avoiding stimulating activities and meals close to bedtime, and having a calm and cosy resting environment are all recommended to help you get better sleep. A more pleasant night's sleep can also be facilitated by easy techniques like utilising blackout curtains, lowering noise levels, and maintaining a comfortable bedroom temperature.

Last but not least, social interaction is essential for controlling dementia. Maintaining social interaction enhances mental health, lessens feelings of isolation and loneliness, and preserves cognitive performance. It is imperative to promote social engagement and meaningful interactions among those diagnosed with dementia.

In order to promote social participation, family members and caregivers can be very helpful. A happy social life can be achieved by organising frequent get-togethers, extending invitations to friends and family, and promoting participation in neighbourhood events.

Making these lifestyle changes may seem overwhelming at first, but with the correct help and direction, they may become a crucial component of managing dementia. I have put together a team of professionals from various wellness and health sectors to assist patients and their families in navigating the obstacles. In addition to counselling and psychology-related procedures, our team offers complete care that includes dietary and lifestyle planning, self-care alternatives, and complementary therapies.

In close collaboration with patients, we create customised lifestyle modification programmes that suit their requirements and interests. We take an empowerment-based approach, working with patients and their families to make long-lasting improvements that will improve their quality of life.

To sum up, a major component of managing dementia is changing one's lifestyle. Enhancing mood and behaviour, boosting overall well-being, and improving cognitive function all depend heavily on social interaction, regular exercise, a nutritious diet, and enough sleep. People with dementia can have a higher quality of life and a stronger sense of control over their disease by putting these adjustments into practise. By working together, we are able to give patients the resources and encouragement they require in order to successfully implement these changes into their life.

Managing Behavioral Symptoms

It can be quite difficult to deal with behavioural problems in both dementia patients and their carers. From mild irritation to extreme agitation and violence, they can fluctuate in intensity. It is critical to realise that these behaviours are the outcome of underlying brain alterations rather than deliberate actions. It is feasible to regulate and lessen these problematic behaviours, resulting in a more tranquil and harmonious environment for all parties concerned, with the appropriate tactics and interventions.

Environmental Modifications:

Assessing and altering the person's surroundings to encourage serenity and lessen stressors is one of the first steps in treating behavioural disorders. Minimizing irritation and aggressiveness requires creating a secure and comforting environment. Here are some important changes to the environment to think about:

1. Reduce Noise and Distractions: For those suffering from dementia, loud noises and intense visual stimuli can be overpowering. Keep the atmosphere as peaceful and quiet as you can, and stay away from loud places and television shows. Calming sounds might come from nature noises or soft, soothing music.

2. Clear Walkways and Minimize Clutter: Disorganized areas can exacerbate misunderstanding and annoyance, which can cause agitation. Clear the living area of any debris and keep the passageways free of obstructions. Basic organising strategies, like labelling cabinets and drawers, can also make it easier for people with dementia to find things and less frustrating for them.

3. Ensure Adequate Lighting: People suffering from dementia may become confused and feel disoriented as a result of poor illumination. Make sure the entire living area is well-lit, especially at night, to enhance visibility and avoid mishaps.

4. Create Familiar and Comforting Spaces: Putting up pictures and items you know well might help people feel at ease and familiar. Make a memory wall or scatter sentimental items about the living space to bring back pleasant memories and ease anxiety.

Communication Techniques:

Managing the behavioural symptoms of dementia requires effective communication. Dementia patients may experience irritation and agitation due to their inability to communicate their needs and feelings. It is possible to promote comprehension and reduce problematic behaviours by employing targeted communication strategies. Several tactics to think about are as follows:

1. Use Simple and Clear Language: Use short, straightforward words and speak slowly and clearly. Steer clear of abstract or difficult concepts. To help with comprehending, break up instructions or inquiries into smaller, more accessible chunks.

2. Maintain Eye Contact and Non-Verbal Cues: People with dementia might feel heard and understood when eye contact is made and non-verbal signs like body language and facial expressions are observed. To foster a relaxing environment, act composed and kind when interacting with others.

3. Validate Emotions: A wide range of emotions can be experienced by people who have dementia. Even if you are unable to completely comprehend or deal with the underlying cause, validate their emotions and acknowledge their feelings. Providing consoling and sympathetic comments might help defuse tense circumstances.

4. Use Visual Aids: Use written instructions or graphics as visual aids to supplement spoken communication. One way to assist people comprehend and adhere to routines is by providing a visual plan of daily activities. This can help people feel less confused and frustrated.

Behavior Management Strategies:

Behavior management techniques, together with communication tactics and contextual adjustments, are essential in the management of behavioural symptoms related to dementia. These techniques concentrate on politely and compassionately rerouting and defusing problematic behaviours. Here are some tactics for behaviour management to think about:

1. Identify Triggers: Keep an eye out for any particular triggers that might be causing the problematic behaviours, and note them. These could be interactions, specific activities, or elements of the surrounding environment. To stop such incidents in the future, try to remove or alter these triggers once you've found them.

2. Distraction and Redirection: If the person becomes agitated or aggressive, divert their focus to another task or subject. Redirecting their attention and reducing tension can be accomplished by assigning them a fun or interesting task.

3. Validate and Redirect: When the person engages in challenging behaviours, acknowledge their feelings and refocus the conversation or activity instead of confronting or arguing with them. For example, if someone becomes upset when doing personal hygiene tasks, try focusing their attention on a happy, comfortable memory.

4. Promote Independence and Autonomy: Encouragement of independence-promoting activities can help reduce frustration and helplessness experienced by people with dementia. To preserve their sense of autonomy and self-worth, provide them the support they need while letting them make their own decisions.

Recall that treating behavioural problems linked to dementia calls for tolerance, comprehension, and a multifaceted strategy. It is imperative to customise interventions to meet the unique needs and preferences of each individual. Speaking with a healthcare expert or dementia specialist might offer specialised direction and assistance all along the way. It is feasible to improve the general wellbeing and quality of life for dementia patients and their carers by using the appropriate techniques.

Caregiver Support and Education

Case Study:

I want to use the case of a patient I recently saw in my medical practise to highlight the need of caregiver education and support. With an early-stage Alzheimer's diagnosis, Mr. Michael Thompson (name withheld for privacy) was a loving husband and caregiver to his wife, Emily.

Mr. Thompson appeared emotionally spent and overburdened when he initially arrived at my clinic. He talked about how hard it was to control his wife's symptoms, which included agitation, confusion, and memory loss. Although he had always been Emily's rock, the responsibilities of being her caregiver were wearing him down.

I stressed the value of caregiver education and support during our first meeting. I clarified that, in his role as a caretaker, Mr. Thompson needed to put his own physical and mental well-being first in order to take good care of his wife. I suggested a comprehensive strategy that would address several facets of his wellbeing, such as support groups, self-care, and short-term care.

Self-Care:

The value of self-care was among our initial discussion topics. I told Mr. Thompson that if he looked after himself, he would be a better caregiver. This required taking good care of his physical well-being through consistent exercise, a healthy diet, and adequate sleep. The importance of emotional health was also underlined, and I offered strategies like journaling, meditation, and reaching out for social support.

In order to help Mr. Thompson put these self-care practises into practise, I put him in touch with a wellness coach who specialises in supporting caregivers. In close collaboration with Mr. Thompson, the coach developed a customised self-care regimen that included enjoyable activities and enhanced his general well-being. Mr.

Thompson was able to enhance his own well-being and more effectively manage the difficulties of providing care by placing a high priority on self-care.

Respite Care:

Respite care was a crucial component of caregiver assistance. I told Mr. Thompson that in order to prevent burnout, it's critical to take regular pauses from providing care. Allowing a professional caregiver or another person to temporarily take over the caregiving duties is known as respite care. You can do this for several hours, a day, or even longer.

I collaborated closely with Mr. Thompson to identify a respite care provider who he felt comfortable with, acknowledging his apprehensions about entrusting his wife to someone else's care. He had to have complete faith in the person watching for Emily while he took his breaks. Together, we were able to locate a reliable respite care provider with a focus on dementia care and staff members with the requisite experience to offer the help and support that was required.

Support Groups:

Joining a support group is an essential part of education and assistance for caregivers. I told Mr. Thompson that making connections with people who were experiencing like things could offer priceless emotional support in addition to helpful guidance. It can also be inspiring and reassuring to hear about the experiences of those who have handled the difficulties of caregiving.

I helped Mr. Thompson get connected with a local support group for dementia caregivers. The group got together on a regular basis to talk about difficulties, impart advice, and exchange experiences. Mr. Thompson was able to establish connections with people in this setting who genuinely recognised the special challenges associated with caring for a person suffering from dementia. It provided him with a safe haven where he could freely express his feelings without fear of repercussion and get advice from people who had been there before.

Mr. Thompson learned about many community resources, services, and caring techniques through his participation in the support group. In addition, he developed sincere relationships with other caregivers, building a network of support for both his spouse and himself.

Conclusion:

The storey of Mr. Thompson is a compelling illustration of how education and support for caregivers may greatly enhance the wellbeing of both the dementia patient and the caregiver. Through prioritising self-care, pursuing respite care, and engaging in support groups, caregivers can enhance their ability to manage the day-to-day issues they encounter.

Prioritizing the well-being of caregivers is vital since they are crucial collaborators in the management of dementia. It is our duty as medical practitioners to make sure caregivers have access to the assistance and information they require. These techniques will help us empower caregivers like Mr. Thompson to give their loved ones the greatest care possible while also taking care of themselves. Add them into our dementia management approach.

Complementary and Alternative Therapies

The area of healthcare has evolved over time to adopt a more holistic approach in addition to standard medical interventions. Alternative and complementary therapies are becoming more and more well-liked as effective ways to treat a variety of illnesses, including dementia. These therapies, which emphasise boosting general well-being, encouraging relaxation, and strengthening cognitive function, are intended to supplement traditional medical treatments.

Aromatherapy is one such treatment. Essential oils derived from plants are used in aromatherapy to enhance mental and physical health. Smell and the limbic system of the brain, which handles memories and emotions, are closely related. It has been discovered that several essential oils offer elevating, soothing, and memory-improving properties.

Aromatherapy can be used to reduce agitation, anxiety, and sleep difficulties associated with dementia. For instance, lavender is well-known for its relaxing qualities and has been demonstrated to lessen agitation in dementia patients. Orange and lemon essential oils, in particular, offer uplifting properties that help improve mood and lessen symptoms of depression. Studies have shown that peppermint oil enhances cognitive performance, especially while doing tasks that call for prolonged concentration and attention.

Another complementary therapy that has demonstrated promise in the treatment of dementia is acupuncture. Acupuncture, a branch of traditional Chinese medicine, is the insertion of tiny needles into particular body locations to promote the flow of qi, or energy. According to studies, acupuncture may aid dementia patients with their memory, cognitive function, and general quality of life.

Acupuncture has been demonstrated in studies to improve blood flow to the brain, which may enhance cognitive function. Additionally, it might have neuroprotective properties that shield brain tissue from deterioration. Furthermore, acupuncture has been shown to lessen anxiety and stress, which are frequently increased in dementia patients. Acupuncture can improve general cognitive function and quality of life by encouraging relaxation and a sense of well-being.

In the field of complementary and alternative therapy for dementia, herbal supplements offer yet another option that merits investigation. Research has indicated that a few herbs and botanicals may be beneficial for overall brain health and cognitive performance. One well-known herb with a reputation for improving memory is ginkgo biloba. It has been extensively researched in relation to dementia and has demonstrated encouraging outcomes in terms of enhancing cognitive function, particularly in those with mild to severe Alzheimer's disease.

Ayurvedic medicine has long employed another herb, Bacopa monnieri, to improve cognitive and memory function. Its efficiency in enhancing memory recall and lowering symptoms of anxiety and depression has been validated by scientific study. The adaptogenic herb ashwagandha has also been linked to a decrease in cognitive decline and an improvement in general brain function.

It's important to recognise the limitations of complementary and alternative therapies, even though they may be beneficial for people with dementia. Further research is required to determine their safety and long-term consequences, as the evidence supporting their efficacy is still developing. Before adding these therapies to a dementia management strategy, as with any treatment, it is imperative to speak with a medical practitioner.

Furthermore, it's critical to address complementary and alternative therapies as a component of an all-encompassing dementia care strategy. These therapies ought to supplement rather than replace traditional medical care. Optimization of general well-being and cognitive performance also requires incorporating lifestyle improvements, such as frequent exercise, a good diet, and stress management.

To sum up, complementary and alternative therapies present viable opportunities to improve the quality of life and cognitive abilities of dementia patients. Acupuncture, herbal supplements, and aromatherapy are just a few of these treatments that may be beneficial. To make sure these therapies are safe and suitable, it's crucial to use caution when using them and to speak with a healthcare provider. Individuals with dementia may see improvements in their general quality of life and cognitive function by including these therapies into a complete dementia management plan.

Palliative Care and End-of-Life Planning

I have personal experience with the difficulties that people with dementia and their families encounter as the illness worsens. I am a medical doctor and health and wellness consultant. In order to guarantee that these people get the assistance they require in their later phases of life, palliative care and end-of-life planning are essential.

The management of dementia requires advance care planning. In order to make decisions about their future medical treatment, individuals must choose a healthcare proxy who will speak on their behalf in the event that they are unable to do so for themselves. It is imperative that those suffering from dementia participate in this process as soon as possible, while their ability to make educated decisions is still intact.

In my practise, I support advance care planning conversations with clients and their families in close collaboration. We analyse the person's values, preferences, and ambitions by delving into a variety of scenarios. In order to customise their care, it is critical that we have candid and open discussions about the things that are most important to each individual. We uphold the autonomy of the dementia patient and guarantee that their desires are carried out by incorporating them in the decision-making process.

Managing symptoms is yet another essential component of palliative care for dementia patients. People may encounter a variety of symptoms as the illness worsens, including pain, agitation, and sleep difficulties, all of which can negatively affect their quality of life. To guarantee comfort and wellbeing, it is crucial to treat these symptoms as soon as possible and in an efficient manner.

To provide thorough symptom management for people with dementia, I work with a multidisciplinary team of professionals from a range of health and wellness domains. Medication modifications, non-pharmacological therapies like aromatherapy or music therapy, and holistic methods like massage or acupuncture may all be part of this. Our goal is to decrease drug use and enhance overall well-being through a holistic approach to symptom management.

Support on an emotional level is essential for people with dementia and their family. All parties involved may experience severe emotional suffering due to the degenerative nature of dementia. As they struggle to remember and speak, people with dementia may feel frustrated, anxious, or depressed. In contrast, caregivers could experience feelings of isolation, exhaustion, and overwhelm in their work.

I provide psychology and counselling to people with dementia and their families in order to help them deal with these emotional issues. When it comes to reducing emotional discomfort in dementia patients, cognitive-behavioral therapy and mindfulness-based therapies have demonstrated encouraging outcomes. Furthermore, support groups and caregiver education initiatives can offer families navigating the challenges of dementia care much-needed emotional support and useful direction.

It is critical to create a support network within the community in addition to the emotional assistance offered by medical professionals. Making connections with other families that are facing comparable challenges can give one a feeling of acceptance and comprehension. For people with dementia and their family, support groups or online forums can be tremendously helpful places to share stories, give and receive advice, and feel less alone.

Though it is a very private and delicate subject, end-of-life planning is necessary to guarantee that people with dementia receive the right care in their last moments. Healthcare professionals and families can make more educated judgments if they have conversations about end-of-life preferences, which include choices on artificial feeding and hydration, life-sustaining therapies, and resuscitation.

I also recommend families and individuals with dementia to think about drafting a living will or advance directive as part of the end-of-life planning process. In the event that the patient loses the ability to express their desires, these documents serve to clarify the patient's preferences for medical care and offer direction to healthcare professionals. Regular reviews and updates are necessary to make sure that these records accurately reflect the person's current preferences.

In conclusion, two essential elements of managing dementia are palliative care and end-of-life planning. Individuals with dementia and their family can receive the necessary care and assistance during their latter stages of life by participating in advance care planning, managing symptoms, and offering emotional support. In order to respect the person's autonomy and make sure their desires are carried out, it is crucial to approach these discussions with kindness, understanding, and dignity. Together, we can successfully manage the challenges associated with dementia care and offer individuals living with this difficult condition all-encompassing support.

Future Directions in Dementia Research

I have devoted many hours to researching dementia research and keeping up with the most recent developments in the field as a medical doctor and health and wellness coach. To give dementia patients the best treatment possible, it is imperative to comprehend the current status of research. I will explore the fascinating field of prospective future directions in dementia research in this subchapter, providing you with a preview of the possible discoveries that may be forthcoming.

The creation of novel treatment options is among the most promising fields of dementia management research. Medication is already available to treat memory loss and cognitive decline, two signs of dementia. The underlying causes of dementia, such as Alzheimer's disease, are still incurable. To find novel therapies that can impede or even reverse the course of these illnesses, researchers are devoting their lives to their research.

The creation of medications that alter disease is one potential advancement in therapeutic choices. The underlying causes of dementia, such as tau tangles and amyloid plaques in the brain, are the targets of these medications. It is believed that the accumulation of these harmful proteins can be decreased, so slowing or perhaps stopping the disease's growth. The effectiveness of these medications is presently being tested in a number of clinical trials, and the preliminary findings are encouraging.

The use of non-pharmacological therapies is another field of research that has a lot of promise for managing dementia. These interventions aim to enhance the cognitive function and quality of life of dementia patients by focusing on lifestyle changes such as nutrition, exercise, and cognitive stimulation. Regular physical activity can both lower the likelihood of acquiring dementia and slow its course in individuals who already have it, according to studies. Moreover, playing brain games and solving puzzles are examples of cognitively stimulating activities that can support the preservation of cognitive function in dementia patients.

Furthermore, the function of nutrition in managing and preventing dementia is being investigated by researchers. A increasing body of research indicates that specific nutrients and dietary styles, such the Mediterranean diet, may help prevent cognitive deterioration and lower the risk of dementia. These discoveries have prompted the creation of customised diets for dementia sufferers, like the MIND diet, which blends aspects of the DASH and Mediterranean diets. To completely comprehend the possible advantages of these dietary changes in the management of dementia, more research is required.

Dementia management also heavily depends on early detection. These days, cognitive tests and clinical symptoms are frequently used to make diagnoses. But by the time symptoms appear, the brain may already have suffered substantial harm. These days, research is concentrated on creating early detection techniques that are more sensitive and accurate.

Utilizing biomarkers, which are quantifiable markers of biological processes occurring within the body, is one such technique. Biomarkers, which include blood levels of particular proteins or structural alterations in the brain as shown by neuroimaging scans, can offer important insights into the onset and course of dementia. Finding these biomarkers may make it feasible to identify dementia early on, enabling earlier interventions and possibly more successful therapies.

Researchers are looking into the use of machine learning algorithms and artificial intelligence (AI) in addition to biomarkers to help in the early detection of dementia. These algorithms can find trends and forecast the chance of getting dementia by analysing vast amounts of data, including brain scans and medical information. Better outcomes for dementia patients could result from increased early detection rates and a change in the field of dementia research thanks to this technology.

Another area of interest in dementia research is enhancing the quality of life for those who have the disease. Cognitive function is frequently compromised by dementia, which can have a major influence on independence and day-to-day activities. To support people with dementia in retaining their cognitive abilities and continuing to participate in meaningful activities, researchers are investigating a range of therapies.

Cognitive rehabilitation is one such strategy that uses focused training and exercises to enhance cognitive function. These therapies can improve a person's overall quality of life by helping a person suffering from dementia regain lost skills and adjust to their cognitive limitations. Psychosocial therapies, such counselling and cognitive-behavioral therapy, can also offer dementia patients and their carers important coping mechanisms and support.

An important factor in raising the quality of life for those suffering from dementia is technology. Wearable technology and smart home technology are two examples of assistive equipment that can help people with dementia preserve their safety and independence. These gadgets can help people with everyday chores, track their location, and serve as prescription reminders. Virtual reality technology is also being investigated as a means of improving cognitive performance and offering immersive experiences that arouse the senses and improve general wellbeing.

In conclusion, there could be significant advancements in dementia care in the near future. Researchers are expanding our knowledge and treatment choices for dementia, from disease-modifying medications and non-pharmacological therapies to early detection techniques and interventions to improve quality of life. I am thrilled to be a part of this quickly developing field as a medical doctor and health and wellness coach, and to help people with dementia and their families on their path to optimum health and well-being.

Chapter 3: Holistic Approaches to Dementia Management

Mindfulness and Meditation

Definition and Context:

The tremendous advantages of mindfulness and meditation for mental, emotional, and physical well-being have made these age-old practises very popular in recent years. The deliberate practise of paying attention just to the present moment, without bias or attachment, is known as mindfulness. It is practising active awareness of one's thoughts, feelings, and experiences as they emerge and bringing the attention back to the here and now with gentleness. Conversely, meditation is an organised technique designed to teach the mind how to attain a heightened awareness and a deep level of relaxation.

The advantages of mindfulness and meditation are especially significant when it comes to dementia. Dementia patients face tremendous obstacles related to memory loss, emotional difficulties, and a steady deterioration in cognitive function. These issues frequently result in elevated stress levels and a weakened sense of overall wellbeing. But by enhancing general wellbeing, reducing stress, and bolstering cognitive function, mindfulness and meditation practises might provide a glimmer of hope.

Enhancing Cognitive Function:

Studies have indicated that consistent mindfulness and meditation techniques help improve cognitive performance in dementia patients. Focus, attention, and concentration are all enhanced by these techniques, which teach the mind to be completely aware of the present moment. Exercises in mindfulness and meditation can also assist people with dementia integrate and absorb information more effectively, which can enhance memory and cognitive processing speed.

The body scan meditation is one such practise that can improve cognitive performance. People are instructed to focus their attention on different bodily parts during this meditation, observing any sensations or feelings that surface. People with dementia can strengthen their general cognitive function by completing this exercise on a daily basis, as it helps them focus and sustain attention.

Managing Stress:

The difficulties and uncertainties related to dementia sometimes result in elevated levels of stress and anxiety. On the other hand, mindfulness and meditation can give dementia patients useful tools for stress management and emotional wellbeing. Studies have indicated that engaging in these activities triggers the body's relaxation response, resulting in a decrease in stress hormone levels and an overall feeling of peace and quiet.

The loving-kindness meditation is a helpful method for managing tension during meditation. This practise entails treating oneself and other people with love and compassion. People with dementia can reduce stress and enhance their emotional health by practising love and kindness. Furthermore, it has been discovered that mindfulness-based stress reduction (MBSR) programmes, which integrate meditation and mindfulness with other stress-reduction methods, considerably lower stress levels in dementia patients.

Promoting Overall Well-being:

Mindfulness and meditation activities improve the general well-being of people with dementia in addition to helping them manage stress and improve cognitive performance. Through these activities, people can cultivate a greater sense of self-awareness and self-compassion by practising active awareness and accepting others without passing judgement. Consequently, this leads to elevated self-worth and an amplified sense of direction and contentment.

Eating mindfully is a practise that enhances general wellbeing and is especially helpful for those who have dementia. This entails paying close attention to the flavour, texture, and experience of the food while eating, as well as being completely present and mindful. People with dementia who practise mindful eating can enhance their digestion, have a better relationship with food, and be less likely to overeat or undereat.

Guided Meditation Exercises:

People suffering from dementia can benefit from mindfulness and meditation by participating in tailored guided exercises. These exercises guarantee that people can simply follow along and reap the advantages of these activities by providing step-by-step instructions and support.

The breath-focused meditation is one such guided practise that has been shown to be beneficial. People are told to concentrate on their breathing during this exercise, paying attention to how the breath feels entering and exiting the body. People who do breathing exercises can develop a state of calmness and serenity and learn to return their focus to the present moment when their thoughts stray.

As previously noted, the body scan meditation is another type of guided exercise. In this activity, every body part is systematically scanned from head to toe, and any feelings or sensations that arise in that body part are noted. The practise of guided imagery, in which people follow a set of instructions for mental visualisation, has been shown to help people unwind and reduce stress.

Conclusion:

For those suffering from dementia, mindfulness and meditation are effective strategies for stress reduction, cognitive function improvement, and general wellbeing. Through these activities, people can strengthen their resilience, become more self-aware, and find serenity even in the face of dementia's obstacles. Moreover, guided meditation exercises offer useful methods that are simple to adopt into everyday schedules, enabling people with dementia to benefit from these practises. Given that every person is different, it is crucial to modify these procedures to accommodate the particular requirements and capacities of dementia patients. People with dementia who practise mindfulness and meditation can go on a self-discovery journey and find peace and comfort in the midst of the complicated realities of their disease.

Nutritional Strategies for Brain Health

Omega-3 Fatty Acids: Superheroes for Your Brain

Let us explore the remarkable advantages of omega-3 fatty acids first. Your brain is shielded from oxidative stress and inflammation by these vital lipids, which act as superheroes for it. Omega-3 fatty acids, especially docosahexaenoic acid (DHA) and eicosapentaenoic acid (EPA), have been linked to improved brain function and may even help prevent dementia, according to a number of studies.

Specifically, DHA is a structurally significant portion of the brain and necessary for the best possible cognitive function. It fosters synaptic plasticity, supports neuronal growth and maintenance, and improves brain connectivity all around. Conversely, EPA can guard against neuronal injury and has strong anti-inflammatory qualities.

Fatty fish, like salmon, mackerel, and sardines, are great sources of DHA and EPA and can help you increase the amount of omega-3 fatty acids in your diet. Alpha-linolenic acid (ALA), which is found in plant-based foods like walnuts, chia seeds, and flaxseeds, can be transformed by the body into DHA and EPA, albeit the process is not as effective as ingesting DHA and EPA straight.

Antioxidants: The Brain's Defense System

Antioxidants are another essential component of your diet for brain health. These potent compounds neutralise free radicals and stop cellular damage, functioning as the brain's defence mechanism. Highly reactive chemicals known as free radicals can lead to oxidative stress, a process linked to ageing and neurological illnesses like dementia.

Studies have indicated that eating a diet high in antioxidants can help prevent cognitive decline and postpone the onset of dementia. Selenium, vitamin C, vitamin E, and flavonoids are a few notable antioxidants.

It has been demonstrated that vitamin E, an important fat-soluble vitamin, reduces oxidative stress and guards against neural damage.

Avocados, spinach, nuts, and seeds are all great food sources of vitamin E.

Water-soluble antioxidant vitamin C is essential for preserving normal brain function. Vitamin C is found in abundance in citrus fruits, berries, bell peppers, and leafy greens, all of which support a healthy, strong brain.

The trace mineral selenium functions as a potent antioxidant and guards against oxidative damage. To enhance the health of your brain, include foods high in selenium in your diet, such as eggs, seafood, Brazil nuts, and whole grains.

Fruits, vegetables, and whole grains include a broad class of polyphenolic chemicals called flavonoids, which have potent anti-inflammatory and antioxidant qualities. Flavonoids are abundant in citrus fruits, dark chocolate, berries, and green tea, and they can improve the health of your brain.

Dietary Recommendations: The Love Language of Your Brain

Adopting a well-rounded and balanced diet is essential to maximising the benefits of nutrition for brain function. Here are some food suggestions that may act as your brain's "love language":

1. Embrace the Mediterranean diet: A lower risk of dementia and cognitive decline has continuously been linked to the Mediterranean diet. While reducing red meat, processed foods, and saturated fats, it places a strong emphasis on whole grains, vegetables, fruits, legumes, nuts, fish, and olive oil. You may feed your brain a lot of nutrients, good fats, and antioxidants by adhering to this eating plan.

2. Prioritize fruits and vegetables: Your brain is drawn to colourful fruits and veggies because they are vivid allies. They include antioxidants and phytochemicals that are critical to preserving brain health. Incorporate as many different hues as you can into your diet each day by including things like cruciferous veggies like broccoli and cauliflower, berries, leafy greens, and bell peppers.

3. Opt for lean proteins: It's critical for brain health to include lean proteins in your diet. Pick lean meats, seafood, poultry, and low-fat dairy items as your sources. These supply vital amino acids that are necessary for the synthesis of neurotransmitters and proper brain function in general.

4. Incorporate whole grains: Whole grains are high in fibre and give your brain steady energy. Examples of these are quinoa, brown rice, and oats. Additionally, they include B vitamins, which are critical for mood and cognitive function.

5. Healthy fats are your friends: Despite having a poor image, healthy fats are essential for maintaining brain function. Add sources of polyunsaturated fats like flaxseeds, walnuts, and fatty fish, as well as sources of monounsaturated fats like olive oil, avocados, and almonds. These fats encourage the best possible functioning of the brain by supporting the composition and structure of brain cells.

6. Hydration is key: Remember how important it is to drink enough of water. Drinking eight glasses of water a day is recommended as it is necessary for optimal brain function. In addition to helping you stay hydrated, herbal teas and infused water provide other health advantages.

Recipe Ideas: Nourishing Your Brain, One Bite at a Time

To help you incorporate these brain-loving nutrients into your daily routine, I would like to share a few recipe ideas:

1. Omega-3 Packed Salmon Salad: For an omega-3 boost, serve baked or grilled salmon with a mix of leafy greens, vibrant veggies like cherry tomatoes and bell peppers, and a dash of flaxseed. For extra taste and lipids that are good for the brain, drizzle with a lemon-tahini dressing.

2. Antioxidant-rich Berry Smoothie Bowl: For a nutrient-dense start to the day, blend a mixture of berries (strawberries, raspberries, and blueberries) with spinach, almond milk, and a tablespoon of nut

butter. For a crunch packed with antioxidants, add chia seeds, walnuts, and a dash of dark chocolate on top.

3. Mediterranean Quinoa Salad: Once the quinoa is cooked, combine it with tomatoes, cucumbers, feta cheese, olives, and a splash of lemon juice and olive oil. This vibrant and tasty salad has the ideal ratio of lean proteins, good fats, and antioxidants that support the brain.

Conclusion:

Adopting brain-healthy eating practises can provide you the ability to prevent dementia by being proactive. Including antioxidants, omega-3 fatty acids, and other nutrients that are good for the brain in your diet will help you maintain good cognitive health and brain function. Keep in mind that your brain deserves the finest, so feed it healthful foods to reap the benefits of increased mental vigour and clarity.

Physical Exercise and Brain Health

Although the many advantages of physical activity for general health have long been known, its effects on cognitive performance and brain health are sometimes overlooked. I will discuss the amazing benefits of exercise for maintaining brain health and cognitive function in dementia patients in this subchapter. I'll go over several exercise modalities, such as strength training and aerobic exercise, and offer helpful advice for fitting exercise into everyday schedules.

Exercise is a strong weapon when it comes to brain health. Regular physical activity has been repeatedly demonstrated to dramatically lower the risk of cognitive decline and postpone the onset of dementia. Exercise is advantageous because it increases neuroplasticity—the brain's capacity to create new connections and adjust to novel experiences—as well as cardiovascular health and blood flow to the brain.

Exercises that are aerobic in nature, like cycling, swimming, or walking, are especially beneficial for brain function. Our heart rates rise during aerobic exercise, which increases the amount of oxygen and nutrients that reach the brain. By strengthening already-existing blood arteries and encouraging the formation of new ones, this process enhances brain function as a whole. Furthermore, cardiovascular activity causes the release of neurotransmitters that are known to improve mood and cognition, such as dopamine and serotonin.

Strength training exercises are just as important for preserving brain function as aerobic activity. People with dementia who participate in resistance-training exercises, including weightlifting or resistance band exercises, can improve both their cognitive and physical capacities. Strength training encourages the brain's production of growth factors, which support the development and upkeep of neurons. Thus, improved memory, focus, and problem-solving abilities result.

Let's talk about how to include physical exercise into our daily routines now that we are aware of the benefits it offers for brain health. It's critical to keep in mind that physical activity doesn't have to be time-consuming or difficult. Simple tasks like cleaning the house or going for a quick walk can have a big impact on brain function.

Start by establishing reasonable objectives for yourself or the dementia-affected loved one. As you get more comfortable, progressively increase the length and intensity of your workouts from short, reasonable beginnings. Selecting activities that suit your physical capabilities and those you love is really important. By doing this, you can make sure that working out becomes a fun and sustainable part of your daily routine.

Making a comprehensive workout schedule might also be beneficial. This plan may include prescribed exercises, such going for a 20-minute walk each morning or performing strength training three times a week. Having a well-organized plan makes it simpler to monitor development and maintain motivation. Furthermore, think about including exercise in your regular routine. To get some extra steps in, you may park further away from your destination or choose to use the stairs instead of the elevator.

In order to augment the advantages of physical exercise on mental well-being, contemplate blending it with additional cognitively stimulating pursuits. Completing puzzles, reading, or picking up a new skill in addition to physical activity might assist optimise the cognitive advantages. By stimulating the brain and encouraging the development of new neural connections, these activities eventually improve cognitive function.

It is important to keep in mind that physical activity should be customised to meet each person's unique demands and capabilities. A healthcare expert should be consulted before beginning any new fitness programme if you or a loved one has any underlying health disorders or concerns. They can offer individualised direction and ensure that the exercise plan is safe and successful.

In conclusion, physical activity is an essential part of managing dementia. By boosting neuroplasticity, increasing cardiovascular health, and inducing the release of neurotransmitters, it supports cognitive function and brain health. It has been demonstrated that strength training and aerobic exercise are especially beneficial for preserving brain health. People with dementia can significantly improve their cognitive capacities by including physical exercise in their regular routines and pairing it with mentally stimulating activities. Recall that even little steps can have a significant impact on your health; physical activity does not have to be time-consuming or difficult. So put on your shoes, make some reasonable goals, and let's go on a trip to improved cognitive function and brain health.

Art Therapy and Creative Expression

A novel approach to treatment, art therapy makes use of several artistic mediums to promote healing and self-discovery. It is an effective instrument that can be used to access the deepest feelings and thoughts of people suffering from dementia, especially in situations where verbal communication becomes difficult.

Painting is among the most researched and successful kind of art therapy for dementia patients. Painting is a visual art form in which people express themselves through images, colours, and shapes that represent ideas and feelings. Studies have demonstrated that painting can improve memory recall by eliciting association memories, particularly when participants are asked to paint scenes from their past or significant life experiences.

Additionally, studies have demonstrated that painting helps enhance dementia patients' communication. Painting serves as a concrete means of communication for people when words fail to convey their emotions and experiences. Making art together with a loved one who has dementia can start a conversation and build relationships that result in meaningful interactions and increased social engagement.

Additionally, it has been discovered that painting improves the emotional wellbeing of those who are suffering from dementia. Painting is a great way to unwind and ease tension and anxiety. It gives people a secure place to express their feelings, which helps lessen the helplessness and frustration that dementia frequently brings with it. Painting can also help people feel more accomplished and confident in themselves since they can see their ideas come to life on the canvas.

Apart from painting, there is evidence that music therapy is beneficial for people suffering from dementia. Even those with late stages of dementia can be moved by the special power of music to arouse memories and feelings. Singing along to well-known songs from their history might bring back memories of important occasions and enhance their mood and general wellbeing.

Moreover, music therapy can improve dementia patients' ability to communicate. Language obstacles can be overcome via the self-expression that comes from singing or playing an instrument. Even in cases where verbal communication is compromised, listening to music can activate brain regions related to speech and language processing. Better relationships with loved ones and social encounters may result from this.

Research has also indicated that artistic pursuits including sculpting, collage, and ceramics can be advantageous for those suffering from dementia. Similar to music and art, these activities help improve communication and trigger memory recall. They provide people a feeling of accomplishment and purpose, which enhances general well-being and a sense of self.

When included into dementia care, art therapy and artistic expression can provide people a sense of empowerment and control over their life. It enables people to stay true to who they are, communicate their needs and feelings, and express themselves. Additionally, these activities can give people a chance to participate in worthwhile and pleasurable activities while serving as a diversion from the difficulties associated with their condition.

The abilities and preferences of the individual must be taken into account when integrating art therapy and creative expression into dementia care. While some people might enjoy painting, others might find happiness and contentment in creating art or playing an instrument. It is recommended that caregivers and healthcare professionals customise the strategy to suit the specific needs and interests of each individual.

To sum up, there are a lot of therapeutic advantages to creative expression and art therapy for people with dementia. Creative pursuits such as painting, music, and other artistic endeavours can boost emotional health, increase communication, and improve memory recall. These types of treatment give people a way to express themselves and help them to keep their sense of self and purpose. The general health and quality of life of individuals with dementia can be improved by integrating art therapy and creative expression into dementia care.

Animal-Assisted Therapy

Animals are used in a special kind of treatment called animal-assisted therapy, or AAT, to help people heal both physically and emotionally. It has shown effective in treating a number of illnesses, such as dementia, anxiety, PTSD, depression, and so on. AAT acknowledges the deep relationship that exists between humans and animals and uses this bond to its advantage to give therapeutic advantages.

The gradual nature of dementia impairs thinking, memory, conduct, and the capacity to carry out daily tasks. For those who are suffering from dementia and their families, it may be a daunting and lonely situation. In my capacity as a physician and health and wellness coach, I am always looking for all-encompassing methods to help my patients live better lives. One such strategy that has showed promise in the treatment of dementia is animal-assisted therapy.

Numerous investigations and studies have demonstrated the beneficial effects of animal-assisted therapy for dementia patients. It has been discovered that having therapy animals around can ease tension and anxiety, encourage relaxation, and even improve cognitive performance. Because they promote socialising and lessen feelings of isolation and loneliness, interactions with animals can have a significant positive impact on one's general well-being.

There are various reasons why animal-assisted therapy for dementia treatment is beneficial. First of all, being around animals can help divert attention from the upsetting signs and symptoms of dementia. They provide solace, company, and an unwavering sense of affection. Animals has a special capacity to provide people with nonverbal assistance and to emotionally bond with people.

Additionally, interacting with therapy animals can improve memory recall and cognitive performance. Petting a dog or cat, for instance, can bring back memories of previous pet ownership or comparable activities. This can create a feeling of identity and connection by igniting discussions and nostalgic experiences. In a similar vein, tending to and feeding animals can provide people a feeling of purpose and accountability, which is especially beneficial for those suffering from dementia.

Emotional and cognitive benefits are not the only advantages of animal-assisted therapy for dementia patients. Benefits to the body have also been noted, such as enhanced motor abilities and bodily functions. One way to fight the physical restrictions that sometimes accompany dementia is to walk or engage with animals. The presence of a therapy animal can serve as a catalyst, inspiring people to lead more active lives and participate in physical activity.

Furthermore, it has been discovered that the use of pharmaceutical interventions in the treatment of dementia is reduced when animal-assisted therapy is employed. Because therapy animals are a natural and efficient way to relax and relieve stress, spending time with them can help cut down on the need for sedative drugs. This is especially important in light of the dangers and adverse effects that this demographic may experience from taking medicine.

The use of animal-assisted therapy in the treatment of dementia calls for some thought and preparation. First and first, it is crucial to protect the therapy animal's health and safety as well as the person suffering from dementia. It's critical to assess the animal's behaviour and temperament as well as the individual's suitability for them. To make sure the therapy is appropriate and successful in these circumstances, collaborating with a trained and certified therapy animal team is crucial.

There are many different kinds of therapy animals, such as dogs, cats, rabbits, and even birds. Every animal has distinct characteristics that may have varying emotional resonances for various people. It's critical to consider the needs and desires of the dementia patient while selecting a therapy animal. The fact that some people may be allergic to certain animals or have animal-related anxieties needs to be taken into account.

In addition, keeping therapy animals in care facilities like nursing homes or memory care units calls for careful supervision and observance of hygienic guidelines. Ensuring the safety and well-being of animals and people they come into contact with requires routine veterinarian examinations, appropriate vaccinations, and infection control protocols.

In conclusion, by lowering agitation, promoting sociability, and raising general quality of life, animal-assisted therapy is a major factor in the management of dementia. The relationship that exists between people and animals is a strong and therapeutic one that has advantages for the body, mind, and emotions. Careful planning and thought must go into implementing animal-assisted therapy to ensure the security and welfare of both the therapy animals and the dementia patients. We can improve the lives of those dealing with dementia by implementing an all-encompassing approach to caregiving. AAT can be a useful tool in the dementia mastery process, offering companionship, comfort, and enhanced wellbeing to those suffering from dementia.

Sleep and Dementia

Our total well-being depends on getting enough sleep, which has an impact on many areas of our health, including memory consolidation and cognitive function. Sleep problems can be especially difficult for those who have dementia, making their symptoms worse and lowering their quality of life. This subchapter examines the complex relationship between sleep disorders and dementia, focusing on how sleep affects memory consolidation, cognitive performance, and general wellbeing. We also offer a comprehensive manual for enhancing sleep hygiene and treating sleep disturbances in dementia patients.

1. Understanding the Link Between Sleep and Dementia:

Sleep is well recognised as being essential to our mental and cognitive functions, memory consolidation, and general well-being. However, this delicate balance can be upset in dementia patients, which can result in a variety of sleep disorders. According to research, people who have dementia are more likely to have disturbed sleep patterns, trouble falling asleep, numerous nighttime awakenings, and excessive daytime sleepiness.

2. Impact of Sleep on Cognitive Function:

There is a complicated relationship between sleep and cognitive function. For the best possible cognitive performance, including attention, concentration, decision-making, and problem-solving, adequate sleep is necessary. Conversely, sleep deprivation damages these cognitive capacities, making it harder for people with dementia to do their everyday responsibilities. Moreover, sleep disturbances might worsen dementia symptoms including disorientation and memory loss.

3. Memory Consolidation and Sleep:

Memory consolidation is the process by which recently learned information is moved and incorporated into long-term memory, and sleep is essential to this process. The brain fortifies the neural connections linked to recently acquired knowledge while you sleep, which improves memory retention. Insufficient sleep can impede this crucial procedure for dementia patients, exacerbating the decline in memory and cognitive abilities.

4. Strategies for Improving Sleep Hygiene in Individuals with Dementia:

a. Establish a Sleep Routine: Better sleep can be encouraged by sticking to a regular sleep pattern, which can assist control the body's internal clock. Establishing a consistent bedtime and wake-up time each day helps help the body link certain times with sleep, which facilitates effortless falling and waking.

b. Create a Relaxing Bedroom Environment: Better sleep can be achieved by creating a relaxing and comfortable sleeping environment in the bedroom. To create a relaxing atmosphere, make sure the space is cold, quiet, and dark. You may also want to try aromatherapy or relaxing music.

c. Limit Stimulants: Sleep disruptions can be avoided by avoiding stimulants close to bedtime, such as caffeine and nicotine. These drugs have the ability to interfere with sleep cycles and make it difficult to get to sleep or stay asleep.

d. Encourage Physical Activity: Frequent physical activity during the day can help you sleep better at night. To prevent overstimulating the body right before bed, it's crucial to plan physical activity for earlier in the day.

e. Implement a Wind-Down Routine: The body can be signalled to relax and get ready for sleep by establishing a wind-down regimen prior to bed. This can involve engaging in relaxing activities like deep breathing exercises or meditation, as well as hobbies like reading a book or having a warm bath.

f. Limit Daytime Napping: The sleep-wake cycle can be upset and difficulty falling asleep at night increased by excessive daytime naps. To reduce their impact on sleep at night, if needed, promote shorter, more regulated naps earlier in the day.

5. Managing Sleep Disorders in Individuals with Dementia:

a. Addressing Insomnia: One of the most frequent sleep disorders in people with dementia is insomnia, which is characterised by trouble sleeping or staying asleep. For this demographic, non-pharmacological therapies like cognitive behavioural therapy for insomnia (CBT-I) can be quite successful in treating insomnia. The main goals of CBT-I include treating the root causes of insomnia, encouraging sound sleeping practises, and enhancing the quality of sleep.

b. Treating Sleep Apnea: Breathing pauses during sleep are a symptom of sleep apnea, which can have a serious negative influence on both the quality of sleep and general health. The gold standard treatment for sleep apnea is continuous positive airway pressure, or CPAP, which may help those with dementia who also have this sleep problem.

c. Managing Restless Leg Syndrome (RLS): RLS, which is typified by an overwhelming need to move the legs, can agitate and disrupt sleep in dementia patients. Medication, lifestyle changes like regular exercise and avoiding triggers like caffeine, and self-help methods like stretching or having a hot bath before bed are all possible forms of treatment for restless legs syndrome.

d. Addressing Nighttime Wanderings: People with dementia frequently wander at night, which can interfere with their sleep cycles and be dangerous. Using tactics like establishing security measures, using nightlights, and creating a safe sleeping environment will help control overnight wanderings and enhance sleep.

e. Managing Sundowning: The term "sundowning" describes a phenomena in which people who have dementia experience increased agitation or confusion in the late afternoon or evening. This may exacerbate insomnia and cause irregular sleep patterns. Sundowning can be controlled by sticking to a daily schedule, reducing outside distractions in the evening, and getting people to do relaxing activities before bed.

In summary, sleep disorders can have a serious negative effect on people who have dementia, aggravating their symptoms and lowering their quality of life. It is essential to comprehend the intricate connection between sleep and dementia in order to develop practical management techniques. We can help people with dementia get better sleep and improve their general well-being by concentrating on enhancing sleep hygiene and treating sleep problems.

Environmental Modifications for Dementia-Friendly Spaces

When creating environments that are dementia-friendly, safety must come first. Dementia causes a cognitive deterioration that makes people more likely to have accidents and injuries because they are less able to manage their surroundings. Thus, it is essential to reduce any risks and establish a safe atmosphere.

Decluttering the living area is a useful strategy for enhancing safety. Not only does removing extraneous furniture, decorations, and other items lessen the chance of falls, but it also de-clutters the space. Simplifying the design of their surroundings can provide people with dementia a sense of clarity and ease, as they frequently struggle with visual and spatial awareness.

Apart from clearing debris, it's a good idea to fasten unsecured carpets, remove any potential trip hazards like cables or wires, and put in handrails in strategic locations. In terms of reducing accidents and encouraging independence, these minor adjustments can have a big impact. Furthermore, you may keep people with dementia from walking off or getting access to toxic chemicals by installing locks on cabinets or doors that lead to potentially dangerous regions, including the garage or basement.

However, environmental changes are not just done to ensure safety. Simplicity is yet another important idea to think about. Dementia patients frequently have trouble making decisions, solving problems, and adhering to complicated directions. Thus, making their surroundings simpler can help them feel less frustrated and anxious.

Putting things in labels and transparent containers is one method to simplify. This makes it simple for people to find their belongings, which can lessen confusion and help people maintain their sense of autonomy. For instance, putting basic labels on kitchen cupboards that list the contents can help someone with dementia feel less anxious about preparing meals.

Setting up visual signals and hints all over the place is also helpful. One way to assist people remember significant dates and keep track of time is to display a large calendar in a conspicuous place. Furthermore, contrasting colour choices for light switches and door handles can help people with vision impairments recognise and operate these objects on their own.

Beyond making sure everything is simple and safe, creating a dementia-friendly setting is important because sensory stimulation improves the quality of life for people with dementia. Using sensory signals and activities to stimulate the senses and support mental and emotional health is known as sensory stimulation.

A good method to elicit happy feelings and enhance the quality of life for individuals suffering from dementia is to include a variety of sensory components. Gently playing background music can trigger memories and improve mood, while soft lighting can produce a serene and tranquil ambiance. Using well-known fragrances, like vanilla or lavender, can also be beneficial and help people relax.

It's critical to offer opportunities for social involvement in addition to sensory stimulation. Dementia patients frequently experience loneliness and social isolation, which can worsen their condition and cognitive abilities. Thus, it's crucial to design areas that encourage social involvement and interaction.

Think about setting up your furniture to promote connection and conversation. Group activities and talks are facilitated when chairs are arranged in a circle or semicircle, as this encourages inclusivity. Establishing spaces set out for socialising and unwinding, such a peaceful garden or a comfortable reading nook, can also promote social interaction and give people a sense of comfort and enjoyment.

Making changes to the home environment is just one part of making spaces dementia-friendly. Supermarkets, dining establishments, and public transit are examples of community spaces that must be modified to meet the special requirements of people living with dementia. Even while big changes might not always be possible, even little adjustments can have an impact.

For example, improving the experience of people with dementia can be substantially increased by teaching employees in public areas how to recognise and accommodate their needs. For individuals with dementia, better navigation and a reduction in anxiety can be achieved by designating quiet spaces, use colours or symbols to denote distinct sections, and having clear signs.

Moreover, integrating dementia-friendly design concepts into newly constructed public areas or structures represents a significant advancement. These guidelines include having high contrast, readily visible fonts on clear signage, reducing reflections and glare, spacing out seating places appropriately, and making sure there are accessible restrooms.

When it comes to making environmental adjustments for dementia-friendly places, it is crucial to remember that there is no one-size-fits-all solution. Because every person with dementia is different and has different needs and preferences, it is crucial to include them in the decision-making process. Their opinions and insights can direct the changes to make sure the setting is customised to meet their unique needs.

In summary, transforming spaces to make them dementia-friendly involves a variety of strategies that centre on social interaction, safety, simplicity, and sensory stimulation. We can help people with dementia feel secure, independent, and well-being by putting these ideas into practise. The ultimate goal is to improve their quality of life and create an environment that promotes their general emotional and cognitive well-being, whether that means making changes to their home or community areas.

Spirituality and Emotional Well-being

When it comes to managing and caring for someone with dementia, it is critical to take their overall wellbeing into account. Addressing mental well-being becomes equally vital as controlling the physical symptoms of dementia, even while medical interventions and therapies are essential. The secret to improving quality of life and building resilience in dementia patients lies in the integration of mental, emotional, and spiritual disciplines.

Dementia patients' emotional health can be a complicated and unstable condition. Dementia-related cognitive impairment frequently causes emotions of annoyance, worry, and terror. People suffering from dementia may experience disorientation and dejection due to their loss of memory and independence, which can lead to a disconnection from their surroundings and sense of self. In this situation, spirituality may be quite helpful in giving people a feeling of direction, significance, and community.

The broadest definition of spirituality is the pursuit of and relationship with something bigger than oneself. This connection can be found in religious practises and beliefs for a great number of people, or it can be experienced through mindfulness, meditation, or a close relationship with nature for others. Whatever its particular shape, spirituality provides a means of reaching within, finding comfort, and achieving a sense of calm and wellbeing.

Facilitating emotional regulation is one of the biggest advantages of integrating spiritual activities into the lives of people with dementia. People with dementia frequently experience increased emotional reactivity, which makes it difficult for them to control their feelings and stay composed. People can reach inner quiet by participating in spiritual practises like prayer or meditation, which offer a calm and centering environment. It efficiently lowers tension and anxiety by enabling individuals to develop a sense of mindfulness and awareness of the current moment.

Particularly, it has been discovered that prayer is a very helpful tool for those suffering from dementia. It provides a direct line of communication with an inner divinity or higher force, providing consolation, comfort, and guidance. Prayer offers people an outlet to communicate their hopes, fears, and anxieties to a higher power during difficult and uncertain times. It fosters emotional resilience and wellbeing by providing comfort and support.

In a similar vein, meditation has shown to be an effective treatment for dementia patients. People can quiet their minds, concentrate on the here and now, and develop self-awareness by practising meditation. It has been demonstrated that meditation lowers anxiety, elevates mood, and increases emotions of general well-being. Meditation offers a sense of calm and shelter in the context of dementia, where patients may experience a constant stream of thoughts and feelings.

Rituals and practises related to religion are also very valuable in helping dementia patients maintain their emotional health. In the face of cognitive decline, the comfortable routines and rituals connected to religious practises might provide a feeling of continuity and stability. They reinforce the concept that one is not alone in one's challenges and provide one a sense of belonging within a community. Furthermore, rituals' spiritual importance gives people a sense of direction and significance, which improves their emotional health.

Beyond the particular exercises listed, a strong feeling of spirituality can be developed in a variety of ways, according to each person's own interests and convictions. Some people use being in nature and fostering a relationship with it as a spiritual practise. Creating art or music is one of the most creative avenues that may be very healing and spiritually gratifying. In the end, it comes down to encouraging people who are suffering from dementia to investigate and adopt spiritual activities that really speak to them.

In summary, spirituality is essential for fostering emotional health and resiliency in dementia patients. Including spiritual activities like meditation, prayer, and religious rituals can help one develop emotional control, access inner resources, and improve one's general quality of life. It is critical for caregivers and medical experts to acknowledge the role that spirituality plays in managing dementia and to make sure that people have access to a wide variety of spiritual activities that can promote their emotional well. By accepting and incorporating spirituality into dementia care, we can provide people the skills and assets they need to face dementia's obstacles with calm, dignity, and emotional fortitude.

Chapter 4: Customizable Plans and Self-Help Techniques

Creating a Personalized Care Plan

There is no one-size-fits-all method when it comes to dementia management. Every person with dementia has different requirements and preferences, and the care plan should take that into account. I will walk you through the process of developing a customised care plan in this subchapter, one that meets the unique needs of both dementia patients and their carers. You can make sure that every facet of their health is taken care of and successfully manage their symptoms by creating a personalised care plan.

Assessing Individual Needs

Performing a comprehensive needs assessment is the first stage in developing a customised care plan. This entails assessing their social, emotional, cognitive, and physical health. It's also critical to get details about their medical background, current prescriptions, and any support networks they may have. I work in conjunction with a range of medical specialists in my practise, such as social workers, psychologists, and occupational therapists, to develop a thorough evaluation of each patient's needs.

Identifying Goals

Establishing the objectives of the care plan is crucial when the assessment is finished. These objectives must to be in line with the person's preferences and wishes, as well as practical and attainable. For instance, if the dementia patient wants to maintain their independence for as long as possible, the care plan should concentrate on putting safety measures in place while still encouraging independence. Together, the dementia patient and their carers can accomplish specific goals by establishing explicit objectives.

Developing Strategies

The following stage is to create plans that address each area of concern found in the evaluation, keeping the goals in mind. This entails taking into account a number of factors, including the administration of medications, physical and mental stimulation, emotional stability, and social interaction. In order to deliver a comprehensive and unique treatment plan, I collaborate with the care team to develop a holistic strategy that incorporates behavioural therapy, lifestyle changes, medicinal interventions, and complementary therapies.

Implementing the Care Plan

It's time to implement the care plan when it has been created. This includes imparting knowledge on the methods and strategies used in the plan to the dementia patient and their carers. It is imperative to guarantee that all parties involved comprehend the reasoning behind every strategy and feel equipped to do the required jobs. Check-ins and follow-up appointments are planned on a regular basis to track progress, address any issues, and modify the treatment plan as necessary.

Evaluating Effectiveness

The process of developing a customised care plan necessitates constant assessment. We can ascertain whether any alterations or revisions to the care plan are necessary by routinely evaluating its efficacy. This entails getting input from the care team, the dementia patient, and their carers. We can make well-informed decisions on the efficacy of the care plan and guarantee that it stays in line with the individual's changing requirements and preferences by aggressively soliciting input from all parties involved.

Personalized Care Plan Templates, Checklists, and Resources

This subsection offers a variety of templates, checklists, and tools to assist people with dementia and their carers in planning and executing their care. Medication schedules, appointments, behavioural observations, and self-care routines can all be managed using these tools. They also act as a reference manual to guarantee that every facet of the care plan is successfully carried out and monitored.

Some examples of the templates and checklists provided in this book include:

1. Medication Log: a thorough journal that assists people in monitoring their drug regimens, dosages, and any side effects. This guarantees that drugs are taken as directed and that any possible problems are quickly resolved.

2. Daily Routine Planner: a visual aid that helps people suffering from dementia keep their sense of regularity and organisation. This planner minimises confusion and lowers anxiety by outlining daily activities, meals, and appointments.

3. Behavior Observation Chart: An instrument for caregivers to track and document any alterations in symptoms or behaviour. The care team can devise effective tactics to tackle these difficulties by using this chart to discover patterns or triggers.

4. Self-Care Checklist: a checklist that motivates people living with dementia to take care of themselves in order to enhance their mental and physical health. This covers pursuits including physical activity, meditation, hobbies, and social interaction.

One can modify these templates, checklists, and resources to suit their own preferences and needs. They act as a guide for planning and directing care, creating channels of communication with the care team, and making sure that every detail of the care plan is taken care of.

Conclusion

For dementia to be effectively managed and the quality of life for the person with dementia and their carers to be improved, a specific care plan must be created. Enhancing an individual's well-being can be achieved by comprehensive assessment, realistic goal-setting, customised strategy development, and care plan implementation. The materials, checklists, and templates in this subchapter are helpful instruments for planning and directing care, encouraging clear communication, and, in the end, assisting in the implementation of a comprehensive strategy for managing dementia.

Cognitive Stimulation Activities

I will give you a range of cognitive stimulation activities in this subchapter that you can include in the everyday routine of people who have dementia. A variety of cognitive levels, interests, and skill levels have been taken into consideration when choosing each exercise. The person with dementia will be more engaged and the potential benefits will be greater if you select activities that are both fun and appropriate for them.

For those suffering from dementia, solving puzzles is a great way to stimulate their cognitive abilities. They are available in a range of shapes and sizes, so you may select the ones that are best suited for the individual you are looking after. Puzzles like Sudoku, word searches, jigsaw puzzles, and crosswords are a few that people with dementia can enjoy. These tasks offer beneficial mental stimulation since they call for the use of problem-solving techniques, focus, and attention to detail.

For those with dementia, memory games are yet another useful cognitive stimulation exercise that can be included in everyday routines. These games have the potential to prevent memory loss, increase cognitive function, and improve memory retention. Simple memory games are entertaining and simple to comprehend. One example is matching pairs, where the player must match identical cards. As the person gains experience, more difficult memory games like picture or sequence recall might be introduced.

Exercises involving creative writing offer emotional release and a platform for self-expression in addition to cognitive engagement. These writing tasks can involve poem creation, journaling, or even short storey writing. Writing can help people with dementia because it fosters creativity, memory recall, and language abilities. Encourage the person suffering from dementia to write down their memories, prior experiences, or even just their current feelings and thoughts. In addition to being a therapeutic exercise, this activity gives people a secure space to share their feelings and ideas.

People with dementia may experience happiness and a sense of success when they participate in arts and crafts activities. Fine motor abilities, creativity, and cognitive function are all enhanced by these exercises. For those suffering from dementia, crafts like knitting, painting, colouring, or even basic origami can be entertaining. People that engage in this kind of creative expression are able to concentrate, pay attention to details, and use their imagination. Selecting activities that suit the person's ability and giving them the assistance and direction they require are crucial.

Research has demonstrated that music listening can positively affect people suffering from dementia. Music improves cognitive function and stimulates different brain regions, eliciting emotions and memories. If the person suffering from dementia is able to play an instrument, encourage them to play one of their favourite tunes. Along with improving cognitive performance and giving oneself a release, singing along to well-known songs can also have these benefits. It has been discovered that music therapy improves the general well-being of dementia patients by lowering agitation and anxiety.

For people suffering from dementia, mental exercises such as puzzles, memory games, creative writing, arts and crafts, and music can greatly enhance cognitive function. It's crucial to keep in mind that these exercises ought to be customised to each person's tastes, skills, and interests. Creating a stimulating and pleasurable environment for the person with dementia, encouraging their independence, and improving their general well-being should be the main priorities.

It is essential to provide a quiet and supportive environment for those with dementia, in addition to the previously listed cognitive stimulation activities. The efficiency of cognitive stimulation exercises can be increased by limiting distractions, establishing a regular schedule, and offering positive reward. To obtain individualised advice and suggestions for cognitive stimulation exercises, it is also advisable to speak with a healthcare provider or dementia specialist.

I have seen firsthand the significant positive effects that cognitive stimulation exercises may have on people suffering from dementia in my capacity as a physician and health and wellness coach. Engaging in these activities enhances cognitive function and improves the general health and quality of life for people suffering from dementia. You may provide people with dementia happiness and fulfilment in their daily life, as well as assist them retain their cognitive abilities, by adding these activities into their daily routine.

Emotional Regulation Techniques

Deep Breathing Exercises:

Deep breathing is one of the easiest yet most powerful methods for controlling emotions. Exercises involving deep breathing can help people with dementia relax, lower their tension and anxiety levels, and quiet their minds. Promoting deep, slow breathing can cause the body to go into a natural relaxation state, which lowers blood pressure and heart rate.

Help the person find a comfortable position to sit or lie down so they can practise deep breathing. As they count to four, have them close their eyes and inhale slowly and deeply. Give them a moment to hold their breath before gently letting go and counting back to four. Carry out this procedure multiple times, paying attention to the feeling of the breath coming into and going out of the body.

Relaxation Techniques:

For those suffering from dementia, relaxing techniques can be immensely helpful in addition to deep breathing exercises. These methods serve to reduce tension and anxiety by fostering a sense of peace and quiet. Progressive muscle relaxation, guided meditation, and rhythmic movement are just a few of the relaxation methods that can be tried.

Tensing and relaxing various bodily muscular groups, ranging from the toes to the head, is known as progressive muscle relaxation. This method aids in releasing physical tension, which lessens mental discomfort. After guiding the person through tensing each muscle group for a brief period of time, tell them to release the tension and observe the change in feeling.

With guided imagery, one can use visualisation to conjure up a serene and tranquil mental scene. Urge the person to picture themselves in a tranquil setting, such a lovely garden or a calm beach. Help them to momentarily escape from any emotional upheaval they may be going through by encouraging them to concentrate on the sounds, smells, and sensations connected to this imaginary area.

Moreover, rhythmic motions like soft rocking or swaying can support mental and physical health. Based on the person's mobility, this can be done standing up or in a chair. Tell them to find a rhythm that feels good for them and to move their body in sync with it, taking in the relaxing and soothing effects of the movement.

Mindfulness Practices:

The benefits of mindfulness activities for stress reduction and emotional well-being are becoming more widely acknowledged. Developing a sense of acceptance, non-reactivity, and paying attention to the current moment without passing judgement are all parts of mindfulness. By practising mindfulness, people with dementia can improve their ability to control their emotions by being more conscious of their thoughts, feelings, and sensations.

The body scan is one easy mindfulness exercise that you can do. Help the person close their eyes and focus on their body, beginning at the top of their head and gradually moving down to their toes. Encourage them to observe any tense spots or sensations in each body part without making any judgments or attempts to alter them. Through this practise, people can become more self-aware and learn how to regulate their emotional suffering.

Mindful breathing is another mindfulness exercise that has potential benefits. This entails concentrating on the breath and paying attention to its organic rhythm and flow. Urge people to focus on the feeling of their breath coming into and going out of their bodies, without trying to regulate or alter it. By keeping people anchored in the here and now, this exercise helps people worry and ruminate less.

Coping Strategies:

Last but not least, it's critical to provide coping mechanisms to people with dementia and the people who care for them so they can overcome any obstacles. Coping mechanisms can assist people in adjusting to changing situations, managing stress, and preserving emotional equilibrium.

Journaling is a useful coping mechanism. Encourage people to write down their ideas and feelings in a notebook or journal as a way of expressing themselves. This can act as a channel for people to express their emotions and think back on their experiences, giving them perspective and clarity. Additionally, journaling offers a priceless record of their dementia experience, enabling patients to monitor their feelings and development over time.

Individuals suffering from dementia and those who care for them may find great benefit from attending support groups. Making connections with people who are experiencing comparable things can be a source of support, understanding, and affirmation. In addition to giving people a safe space to talk about their emotions, worries, and experiences, support groups may frequently give insightful counsel and direction.

To sum up, emotional control strategies are crucial to the management of dementia. The implementation of deep breathing exercises, relaxation techniques, mindfulness practises, and coping skills can significantly enhance emotional well-being and facilitate the management of potential issues for both individuals with dementia and their caregivers. People can experience more serenity, better emotional health, and an improved quality of life by adopting these practises into their everyday routines.

Keep in mind that every person's experience with dementia is different, so it could take some time to determine which methods are most effective for them. It is crucial for me to keep investigating and learning new tactics as a healthcare expert in order to guarantee that people with dementia receive comprehensive support and care. By working together, we can enable people with dementia and those who care for them to better handle the emotional effects of the disease and pursue higher standards of living.

Communication Strategies

Effective communication requires listening, which is even more important when speaking with those who have dementia. When conversing with them, it's critical to be really present and give them the opportunity to speak without interjecting. In my experience as a healthcare worker, being attentive and patient can have a profound impact. It gives dementia patients a feeling of agency and affirmation, boosting their sense of self-worth and encouraging effective communication.

In addition, active listening entails focusing on non-verbal indicators like gestures, body language, and facial expressions in addition to hearing what is being said. Even in cases where a person with dementia has little verbal capacity, these signs can frequently offer insightful information about their needs and feelings. In my experience, caregivers and medical professionals can improve communication by paying attention to these non-verbal indicators, which help them better comprehend and address the needs and feelings of the individual.

It is essential to take into account the distinct abilities, strengths, and limitations of individuals with dementia in order to properly modify communication to their cognitive abilities. Since every person's experience with dementia is unique, communication tactics must be adjusted accordingly. While some people could find it difficult to follow long conversations or digest complex information, others might have trouble expressing themselves verbally. Simplifying language and using clear, succinct words are crucial. Jargon and unclear terminology should be avoided as they might cause confusion.

Moreover, conversing with someone one-on-one in a calm and serene setting can significantly improve communication for those suffering from dementia. Reducing outside distractions—like loud background noise or intense visual stimulation—can assist people in maintaining cognitive engagement and attention span during conversations. People can express themselves more freely and an atmosphere of effective communication is fostered as a result.

Using visual aids, such picture cards or gesture clues, can be quite beneficial for people with dementia, as I have discovered in my practise. These tools and suggestions can help with comprehension and communication. When a caregiver is talking to a person who is having trouble expressing their preferences, for instance, pointing to the selections or giving them photographs of various meals can help the person make a clearer decision. Furthermore, by adding context and enhancing spoken cues, gestures can improve communication even further.

Using validation strategies is another helpful communication strategy for people who are suffering from dementia. Recognizing and appreciating someone's emotions entails validating them even when their views or ideas don't match reality. By building rapport and trust with the person, this method seeks to lessen the possibility of resistance or agitation during conversation. Caregivers and medical professionals can establish a secure and supportive environment that encourages open and honest conversation by recognising their emotions and experiences.

Understanding that communication is a two-way street is also crucial. People with dementia should be given the chance to express themselves and actively participate in conversations, even though caregivers and medical experts are crucial in fostering successful communication. Open-ended questions, which permit more detailed answers and motivate people to express their ideas and emotions, can help achieve this. Giving people with dementia options and decision-making chances also gives them a sense of empowerment and maintains their dignity and sense of autonomy in social relationships.

People may find it harder to start or continue discussions as their dementia worsens. It becomes imperative in these situations for caretakers and medical experts to take the initiative and direct the discussion. One effective strategy for having meaningful conversations with people who have dementia is to use recollection therapy. In order to facilitate connection and dialogue, caregivers can ask patients to recall particular past experiences or occurrences. This retains a feeling of self and improves the relationship between the care recipient and the caregiver in addition to promoting cognitive function.

In summary, preserving meaningful connections, fostering well-being, and improving overall dementia management all depend on good communication strategies for people with dementia and their carers. Caregivers and healthcare professionals can establish a pleasant communication environment by using non-verbal cues, active listening, modifying communication strategies according on cognitive skills, and implementing reminiscence therapy and validation. It is imperative to keep in mind that communication is a dynamic process that calls for patience, empathy, and flexibility. By putting these techniques into practise, people suffering from dementia can maintain communication about their needs, feelings, and thoughts, which improves their general quality of life and wellbeing.

Memory Enhancement Techniques

As a physician and health and wellness coach, I have worked with many people who are suffering from dementia and its terrible effects on memory. My desire to discover efficient memory-enhancing methods was stoked by seeing the suffering and annoyance that come with memory loss. I will look at a number of methods in this chapter that can help dementia patients with memory retrieval and retention. These methods, which range from mnemonic devices and memory aides to memory training activities, can offer a comprehensive plan for managing dementia.

Let's start by recognising the difficulties with memory that people with dementia encounter. A neurological condition called dementia impairs cognitive abilities like memory, thinking, and problem-solving skills. Specifically, memory loss can have a major influence on a person's day-to-day functioning by making it difficult to recall names, dates, and even basic chores. On the other hand, we can enable people suffering from dementia to increase their memory and reclaim control over their life by applying memory enhancement therapies.

Mnemonic devices are an effective way to improve memory. Mnemonics are tools for improving memory that help encode knowledge so the brain can access it more easily later. These can be represented in a number of ways, such as chunking strategies, visual aids, and acronyms. To help someone remember a list of things, they can make an acronym out of the initial letter of each item. For example, "ROYGBIV" can help someone recall the colours of the rainbow. By using the brain's ability to recall patterns and associations, this method facilitates the retrieval of knowledge.

On the other hand, memory aids are tangible objects or techniques that help people with dementia recall crucial information. Depending on the needs of the individual, these aids can be basic or complicated. For example, putting sticky notes all over the house to remind people of regular responsibilities can be a simple memory aid. Reminders and other critical information can also be recorded using more complex tools like voice recorders or smartphone apps. By acting as outside cues, these tools help make up for the cognitive deficiencies brought on by dementia by triggering memory recall.

Memory training exercises, in addition to mnemonic devices and memory aides, can greatly enhance memory function in dementia patients. Memory retention can be enhanced and new neural connections can be formed in the brain through the use of memory training exercises, which are specifically designed activities. These exercises can take many different forms, such as playing memory-retrieving games and puzzles or attending memory seminars or programmes run by qualified experts. These activities are intended to improve memory as well as provide dementia patients a feeling of empowerment and success.

Using recognition tasks is one method of memory training. This entails giving someone a series of stimuli, like images or objects, and then asking them to identify them later. This kind of exercise strengthens memory pathways and recall skills by stimulating the brain's capacity to retrieve stored information. Repetition and rehearsal strategies can also be employed in memory training exercises. People with dementia can improve their encoding and retrieval skills, which will help them remember and recall knowledge more successfully, by repeating information.

Additionally, a memory-training method called cognitive stimulation therapy (CST) has demonstrated encouraging outcomes in enhancing memory function in dementia patients. As part of CST, participants engage in group sessions that address a variety of cognitive tasks, including talks, puzzles, and memory treatment. These sessions give dementia patients the chance to interact socially and mentally, two things that have been demonstrated to improve memory. CST also offers a safe space for people to talk about their experiences and get support, which helps people remember things better and retrieve them more easily.

Finally, I must stress the significance of lifestyle changes in improving memory for those with dementia as a holistic healthcare professional. Research has revealed that things such as exercise, good food, and quality sleep can dramatically impact memory performance. Frequent exercise strengthens memory and the cardiovascular system in addition to the brain. Adding mental exercises like yoga, dance, or walking to everyday routines can help with memory retention and brain stimulation. A healthy diet that includes important nutrients like antioxidants and omega-3 fatty acids can also boost brain function and improve memory. Last but not least, getting enough sleep is critical for memory consolidation, which enables the brain to efficiently process and store information.

To sum up, memory improvement methods offer priceless resources for the all-encompassing care of dementia. These techniques give dementia patients a road map for enhancing their memory retention and retrieval, from mnemonic devices and memory aids to memory training activities and lifestyle adjustments. People with dementia can regain control over their memory function by using targeted cognitive tasks, environmental signals, and the brain's ability to make associations. By adopting a comprehensive strategy for managing dementia that encompasses the physical, mental, and emotional aspects of well-being, we can enable people affected by dementia to lead satisfying lives even in the face of the debilitating illness.

Problem-Solving and Decision-Making Skills

I have worked closely with people who have dementia for many years in my medical practise, and I have seen firsthand the significant impact that a decline in their ability to solve problems and make decisions can have on their day-to-day life. These mental skills are essential for independence maintenance, day-to-day task management, and even personal safety. As a result, it's critical to provide dementia patients with the instruments and techniques they require to improve these abilities.

I will walk you through a number of approaches and models in this chapter that have been shown to improve the ability to solve problems and make decisions in people who are suffering from dementia. We'll look at decision-making frameworks, adaptive tactics, and structured problem-solving methods that can aid with cognitive difficulties.

An organised method for recognising and fixing issues is offered by structured problem-solving approaches. These methods have been shown to be beneficial in helping people with dementia decompose difficult issues into smaller, more doable steps.

Finding the problem is the first stage in the structured problem-solving process. Urge those suffering from dementia to express the precise problem they are experiencing or the objective they wish to accomplish. After the issue has been located, it is critical to collect pertinent data. This can be accomplished by having discussions, gathering information, or speaking with authorities in the area.

The process of coming up with possible answers comes next. It is crucial to establish a secure and encouraging environment where people with dementia feel free to communicate their ideas in order to foster creative thinking. Urge them to explore different options and think creatively. Tell them that every input is valuable and that there are no right or wrong responses.

It's time to assess and select the best choice after coming up with various options. Assist those suffering from dementia in weighing the benefits and drawbacks of each option in light of their particular needs and preferences. Help them comprehend the possible outcomes of each choice, both favourable and unfavourable.

Putting the selected answer into action is essential as soon as a decision is made. Divide it into manageable chunks and offer the assistance and direction you need as you go. Urge people suffering from dementia to ask for help from their friends and family or medical experts if necessary.

Additionally useful tools for improving the problem-solving and decision-making abilities of dementia patients are decision-making frameworks. These frameworks offer a methodical and organised way to approach well-informed decision-making. The "Five W's and an H" structure has the following elements: Who, What, Where, When, Why, and How.

With this approach, people suffering from dementia can ask themselves the following questions to help them critically assess a situation or issue:

- Who is involved? Identify the people or organizations that are stakeholders or have influence over the decision.

- What information do I need? Identify the facts, data, and relevant knowledge required to make an informed decision.

- Where should I gather this information? Identify the sources and channels from which information can be obtained.

- When do I need to make a decision? Determine the timeline or deadline by which a decision needs to be made.

- Why is this decision important? Understand the significance and potential impact of the decision on oneself and others.

- How can I implement this decision? Develop a plan of action and identify the necessary resources and support.

People suffering from dementia can make better decisions by methodically analysing and evaluating the issue by answering each of these questions.

Adaptive strategies are essential for helping people with dementia overcome cognitive problems, along with structured problem-solving procedures and decision-making frameworks. These tactics concentrate on making up for cognitive deficiencies and applying other methods for solving problems and making decisions.

Dividing difficult activities into smaller, more doable chunks is one adaptive method. This lowers the cognitive strain and raises the likelihood of success. A home duty that the person with dementia is finding difficult to finish, for instance, can be made more manageable by segmenting it into smaller subtasks and giving step-by-step directions.

Using technologies and external aids is another adaptive tactic. This could involve prompting people with dementia to finish particular chores or make decisions by using smartphone apps, alerts, or reminders. These tools can compensate for memory and cognitive deficiencies and serve as cognitive supports.

Incorporating trustworthy individuals such as family members or caretakers into the decision-making process can yield invaluable insights and assistance. People with dementia can gain from other viewpoints and new knowledge when others are involved in the decision-making process, which will ultimately result in better judgments.

People with dementia can continue to make educated decisions and reclaim a sense of control over their lives by using adaptive tactics, decision-making frameworks, and structured problem-solving techniques. It is important to keep in mind that even though they may have cognitive impairments, they are still capable of making decisions and solving problems. It is our duty as caretakers and medical experts to give them the assistance and resources they need to deal with the difficulties caused by dementia.

We will look at more methods in the upcoming chapter for reducing the symptoms of dementia and enhancing general wellbeing. Through addressing the psychological, social, and physical elements of dementia, we can develop a comprehensive plan for end-to-end care. Follow us as we explore the complex aspects of dementia and find practical methods for enhancing wellness and health in those who have the disease.

Self-Care and Well-being for Caregivers

I know personally the tremendous physical, emotional, and mental toll that providing care can take on people because I work as a health and wellness coach. The requirements of their loved ones with dementia are frequently given priority by caregivers, who give up their time and energy to see to it that their needs are satisfied. But it's critical for caregivers to never forget how vital it is for them to look after themselves. It is possible for caregivers to effectively manage the difficulties of caregiving and preserve their own health and well-being by making self-care a priority and connecting with support systems.

It can be a demanding and stressful experience to provide care, therefore it's critical that caregivers understand and control any stress they may face. Prolonged stress can have a negative impact on one's physical and emotional well-being, raising one's risk of diseases including depression, heart disease, and high blood pressure. The development of coping mechanisms that encourage rest and self-care is essential for the efficient management of caregiver stress.

The use of mindfulness and meditation as stress management techniques is one that works well. Focusing on and accepting the current moment without passing judgement is a key component of mindfulness. Caregivers can foster a sense of calm and lower stress levels by implementing mindfulness into regular tasks. Easy mindfulness practises can have a big impact on lowering caregiver stress. Some examples of these practises are deep breathing exercises and setting aside some time each day for a calming activity.

Keeping up a healthy lifestyle is another crucial component of self-care for caregivers. Regular exercise and a healthy diet can improve resilience to stress and promote general well-being. Because we are time- and emotionally-pressed, it is easy for us to forget about our own nutritional needs and to engage in poor eating habits as caregivers. However, caregivers can increase their energy levels and advance their own well-being by setting aside time for exercise and choosing wholesome food.

Moreover, joyful and calming self-care activities shouldn't be disregarded. Hobbies and other enjoyable pursuits can provide caregivers with a much-needed break from the obligations of caregiving. Finding time to do enjoyable and stress-relieving activities—like painting, gardening, reading, or just taking a stroll in the park—is crucial for caregiver self-care.

Apart from employing self-care techniques, caregivers must to deliberately pursue assistance from others who are undergoing comparable circumstances. Being a caregiver can frequently feel lonely, therefore having other people's support and empathy can be incredibly consoling. Support groups designed especially for those who look after people with dementia can be a great place to get knowledge, inspiration, and emotional support. These organisations allow caregivers a forum to talk about their experiences, get guidance, and build deep relationships with people who genuinely get their path.

Creating a solid support system might encompass family, friends, and medical experts in addition to support groups. It's critical that caregivers ask for assistance when necessary and delegate some of the caregiving duties to others. Sharing the effort can reduce stress and minimise burnout, whether it is through employing professional caregiver services or asking a family member for help with specific duties.

Finally, important components of caregiver self-care include taking pauses and engaging in self-compassion exercises. Understanding that no one can handle everything on their own and that it's acceptable to ask for assistance and take care of oneself is crucial. Caregivers can rest and recharge by taking breaks from their caring duties, which enables them to give their loved ones better care. Taking care of oneself with love and understanding, admitting the difficulties of providing care, and forgiving oneself of flaws and limits are all parts of practising self-compassion. Caregivers who possess self-compassion are able to handle the highs and lows of providing care with dignity and acceptance of themselves.

In summary, when caring for people with dementia, caregivers' health and well-being come first. In addition to maintaining their own physical, emotional, and mental well-being, caregivers can better negotiate the obstacles of caregiving by putting stress management techniques into practise, encouraging healthy living habits, asking for help, and engaging in self-compassion exercises. Caregivers can ensure a more balanced and long-lasting caregiving journey by practising self-care, which allows them to foster a supportive atmosphere for both themselves and their loved ones.

Adapting to Changing Needs and Challenges

A degenerative condition, dementia impairs memory, thinking, and reasoning, among other cognitive abilities. This illness not only affects the patient but also has a significant effect on their loved ones and caretakers. A flexible and dynamic approach to care is necessary when the disease worsens since it changes the requirements and difficulties that the patient and their carers must deal with.

Acknowledging the disease's progressive nature is a first step towards adapting to evolving requirements and problems. Dementia is a dynamic illness that presents differently in every person and advances at their own rate. It is imperative that healthcare providers and carers periodically reevaluate the patient's status and modify the care plan as necessary. This could entail trying out different therapy, introducing fresh approaches, or changing tactics.

Open communication and cooperation between the patient, their caregivers, and medical personnel are necessary when modifying care plans to accommodate evolving needs. It is imperative to conduct periodic assessments of the efficacy of existing interventions and implement requisite modifications to guarantee that the demands of the individual are fulfilled. In order to handle certain difficulties like behavioural problems, medication management, or psychological assistance, this may entail bringing in extra healthcare personnel or specialists.

Adopting novel strategies is equally important for managing dementia as is adjusting care plans. New treatments, methods, and therapies are being created as our knowledge of the illness advances. It is critical to keep up with the most recent findings and developments in dementia care, as well as to be open to considering other treatment options. Investigating cutting-edge technologies like assistive gadgets or virtual reality programmes may be necessary to do this, as well as incorporating complementary therapies like aromatherapy, music therapy, or art therapy into the care plan.

Being open to trying new things also means being prepared to think beyond the box of conventional healthcare models and take a holistic approach to treatment. As a health and wellness coach, I have witnessed firsthand the transforming potential of dietary and activity changes in the management of dementia symptoms. People with dementia can benefit from enhanced cognitive performance, mood, and quality of life by emphasising overall wellness and embracing healthy practises.

Having a thorough awareness of each person's particular requirements and difficulties is essential to managing dementia. Every person with dementia has a unique experience, therefore it's critical to customise the care plan to meet their needs. This could entail taking their cultural background, values, and personal preferences into account. We can better satisfy each person's needs and enhance their general well-being by developing a personalised approach to care.

It is necessary to be flexible and adaptable while creating care plans and treatment plans as well as when interacting on a daily basis with people who have dementia. People may have trouble communicating, remembering things, and controlling their emotions when their cognitive abilities deteriorate. It is essential that caretakers and medical professionals communicate with patience, adaptability, and understanding. This could entail streamlining communication, applying empathy and validation tactics, and making use of visual aids to make people feel heard and understood.

Recognizing that the demands and difficulties of caregivers change along with those of the individual is another crucial component of flexibility in dementia care. Physical, emotional, and mental tiredness can result from caregivers' frequent large time and energy commitments to helping their loved ones. It is crucial for caregivers to put self-care first and ask for help when they need it. To do this, you might want to get in touch with support groups, look for temporary care, or ask other family members or trained caregivers for assistance.

In the end, becoming adaptive to new demands and difficulties is a complex, continuous process. It necessitates a comprehensive strategy that incorporates medical knowledge, compassion, and an openness to considering novel options. Individuals suffering with dementia and their carers can effectively traverse the intricacies of the illness and discover purposeful methods to improve quality of life by adopting an attitude of adaptation and flexibility. A customised, flexible strategy that changes with the demands of the individual is needed for dementia care; there is no one-size-fits-all approach. We can enable people with dementia to live life to the fullest despite the obstacles they encounter by being adaptable and welcoming of new ideas.

Chapter 5: Evidence-Based Insights and Future Directions

Latest Research on Dementia

Millions of people worldwide are impacted by the complicated and multidimensional disease known as dementia. In order to give my patients the greatest treatment and support possible, as a medical doctor and health and wellness coach, I am constantly searching for the most recent findings and developments in dementia management. I'll get into the cutting-edge research that could completely change how we treat dementia in this subchapter.

The discovery of biomarkers is an important field of research in dementia care. Measurable compounds or signs known as biomarkers are useful for tracking the development or diagnosis of diseases. Researchers have come a long way in finding particular biomarkers that can help with early detection in the case of dementia. For instance, the development of Alzheimer's disease, the most prevalent type of dementia, has been connected to the buildup of tau tangles and amyloid-beta plaques in the brain. Additionally, modifications to proteins in the cerebrospinal fluid, such as neurofilament light chain (NfL), have been found in studies to be possible dementia biomarkers. Healthcare providers can diagnose dementia early and provide appropriate therapies and better disease management by identifying these biomarkers.

Additionally, neuroimaging methods have been essential in improving our knowledge and treatment of dementia. Researchers can identify the structural and functional alterations linked to dementia by using precise images of the brain obtained from positron emission tomography (PET) and magnetic resonance imaging (MRI). For example, MRI scans can show atrophy in the brain, whereas PET scans can show lower glucose metabolism in some parts of the brain, which suggests malfunctioning of the neurons. Furthermore, neuroimaging methods can help distinguish between various forms of dementia and improve the accuracy of the diagnosis.

The creation of novel treatment approaches is a fascinating field of study in dementia care. Traditionally, symptom management has been the main emphasis of dementia treatment. But more and more, scientists are looking into cutting-edge methods to curtail or even reverse the disease's course. Clinical trials have demonstrated potential in addressing the underlying pathology of Alzheimer's disease, including tau and amyloid-beta. Aducanumab is one of the monoclonal antibodies that have been created to specifically target and eliminate amyloid-beta plaques from the brain. Though further research is needed to determine the effectiveness of these medicines, they provide hope for future advancements in the treatment of dementia.

Researchers are looking into the possibilities of lifestyle changes and alternative therapies in addition to traditional drugs for the management of dementia. Several studies have demonstrated that a good diet, frequent physical activity, and stimulating cognitive activities can all help lower the risk of dementia and halt its progression. For example, it has been discovered that aerobic exercise helps people with Alzheimer's disease prevent brain shrinkage and enhance cognitive performance. A diet centred around fruits, vegetables, whole grains, and healthy fats, similar to the Mediterranean diet, has also been linked to a decreased risk of dementia. Additionally, a number of complementary therapies have been demonstrated to have a significant impact on the quality of life and overall wellbeing of those diagnosed with dementia, including art therapy, music therapy, and recollection therapy.

In addition, psychological and emotional support are crucial for managing dementia. Dementia frequently causes cognitive decline, memory loss, and behavioural abnormalities in its victims, which can exacerbate their frustration, worry, and melancholy. Thus, improving the general wellbeing of people with dementia and their carers requires the development of efficient coping mechanisms as well as counselling. Relaxation techniques, mindfulness-based therapies, and cognitive behavioural therapy (CBT) have all demonstrated promise in the management of psychological symptoms related to dementia. In a similar vein, caregiver burden can be decreased and mental health can be enhanced by enrolling caregivers in support groups and offering them information and tools.

In conclusion, because of the most recent discoveries and developments, the field of dementia management is always changing. Through the identification of biomarkers, use of neuroimaging techniques, and creation of novel treatment modalities, researchers are making substantial progress toward the development of more efficient methods for dementia diagnosis, management, and therapy. Moreover, lifestyle adjustments, complementary and alternative therapies, and psychological support have been identified as essential elements of dementia care, improving overall health and quality of life. I am dedicated to remaining up to date on the most recent research as a medical doctor and health and wellness coach so that I may offer my patients the most thorough and successful dementia treatment techniques. We can enable people with dementia and those who care for them to face this difficult path with hope and resilience by incorporating these discoveries and knowledge into our approach.

Promising Therapies and Clinical Trials

Millions of people worldwide suffer from dementia, a progressive neurological condition marked by cognitive decline and functional disability. It has been difficult to find effective medicines to stop or reverse the progression of dementia. But new discoveries in medicine have given us optimism for a better tomorrow.

Treatments that modulate the dementia symptoms represent one of the most promising areas of dementia research. In an effort to change the course of the illness and possibly even stop or reverse its progression, these treatments focus on the fundamental mechanisms causing it. To this end, researchers have been experimenting with a number of strategies, such as encouraging neurogenesis and synaptic plasticity and focusing on the accumulation of tau tangles and amyloid-beta plaques in the brain.

Early research on a number of novel medications has shown promise. For example, amyloid-beta monoclonal antibodies, such aducanumab, have shown promise in lowering the amount of amyloid plaque in the brain. This decrease in plaques could slow down cognitive ageing and enhance brain health in general. Similarly, medications that target tau protein aggregation, such as LMTX, have demonstrated promise in lowering tau tangles and maintaining cognitive function. Strict clinical trials are being conducted on these disease-modifying therapies to ascertain their safety and effectiveness.

Another innovative strategy being investigated in the realm of dementia is immunotherapy. The removal of infections and aberrant proteins from the brain is largely dependent on the immune system. But in diseases like Alzheimer's, the immune system can become dysregulated, which can cause long-term inflammation and damage to the neurons. The goal of immunotherapies is to improve the immune system's capacity to eliminate harmful substances like tau and amyloid-beta.

Targeting amyloid-beta by active or passive vaccination is one such immunotherapy. By administering a modified form of amyloid-beta to recipients, active immunisation stimulates the production of antibodies by the immune system against this protein. In contrast, prepared antibodies are given directly to individuals during passive immunisation. By binding to amyloid-beta, these antibodies help the protein to be removed from the brain.

Immunotherapies have been the subject of promising clinical trials. For instance, in people with early-stage Alzheimer's disease, the BAN2401 antibody significantly lowered the load of amyloid plaque and slowed the rate of cognitive loss. Furthermore, the FDA approved the Aduhelm antibody for the treatment of Alzheimer's disease due to its capacity to lower amyloid plaques.

Another promising treatment option for dementia is gene therapy. Through focusing on particular genes implicated in the advancement of the disease, scientists hope to change the way these genes express or function, which will ultimately change how the disease develops. For example, researchers are looking into how the apolipoprotein E (APOE) gene may be involved in Alzheimer's disease. The APOE ç4 allele is one of the gene polymorphisms that raises the risk of the disease.

These genetic variations can potentially be edited or modified by gene treatments like CRISPR-Cas9. Researchers want to lower the chance of Alzheimer's disease in people who are at high risk of getting the disorder by changing or correcting the APOE gene. This is a technique that needs more development before it can be regarded as a practical therapeutic option. But there's no denying that gene therapy has the potential to completely change the way dementia is treated.

Even though there is a lot of promise for these therapies, it is crucial to be cautious and understand that they are still in the experimental stages. Years of extensive testing and clinical trials are necessary before a medication is deemed safe and suitable for general usage. To get these treatments on the market, it's also critical to handle moral dilemmas, guarantee patient safety, and handle regulatory procedures.

In conclusion, those impacted by dementia and their families have hope thanks to the search for effective treatments and the ongoing clinical research in this sector. Gene therapy, immunotherapy, and disease-modifying therapies are just a few of the fascinating directions being investigated in research facilities worldwide. The lives of persons suffering from dementia could be drastically changed by future advances in these fields, notwithstanding the difficult and lengthy search for appropriate therapies. I'm dedicated to remaining on the cutting edge of these developments as a medical professional and health and wellness coach in order to give my patients the greatest treatment and support possible as they progress toward mastery of dementia.

Technology and Dementia Management

In my experience as a medical professional and health and wellness coach, technology has a profoundly positive impact on dementia care. The lives of those with dementia and those who care for them can be greatly enhanced by the creative solutions made possible by technological breakthroughs. This subsection will explore the diverse approaches that technology can employ to improve the care of individuals with dementia.

In order to help people with dementia in their daily lives, assistive technologies have become increasingly important. By compensating for cognitive and functional deficits, these devices help people keep their independence and standard of living. Smart home technology that can be incorporated into a dementia patient's living space is one such instance. Some of the everyday tasks that these devices can help with are medicine reminders, assisting users with getting around the house, and alerting caretakers to emergencies.

Wearable technology has also grown in popularity for managing dementia. These gadgets, which might be smartwatches or bracelets, can track a person's whereabouts and keep an eye on their vital signs, giving comfort to both the person with dementia and their carers. In the event that a dementia patient wanders off or has an unexpected change in their condition, they can also notify caretakers via alerts. This makes it possible to intervene quickly and guarantees the person's safety and wellbeing.

Systems for remote monitoring have also been more crucial in the treatment of dementia. By enabling remote monitoring of an individual's cognitive and functional capacities, these technologies give caretakers and healthcare professionals important new perspectives on their condition. One way to administer cognitive exams remotely is by using telemedicine platforms, which enable people to complete tests from home. This eases the strain of needing to attend the clinic frequently and gives medical experts access to real-time data to help them decide on the best course of therapy for the patient.

Moreover, technological advancements have made virtual reality therapies possible for the therapy of dementia. The potential for virtual reality (VR) to improve cognitive performance and the general well-being of dementia patients has been demonstrated. VR therapies have the potential to enhance cognitive engagement and brain stimulation by submerging participants in a virtual environment. One way that VR games and simulations can help people with dementia is by improving their problem-solving, memory, and attention span. In addition to their therapeutic effects, these therapies provide dementia patients something fun and entertaining to do.

Furthermore, communication for those suffering from dementia has been transformed by technology. Dementia patients may find it difficult to explain themselves or to understand both verbal and nonverbal clues, which can make communication extremely challenging. But there are a number of communication methods available thanks to technology that can close these gaps. For example, spoken words can be converted into written text using computerised speech-to-text software, which makes it easier for people with dementia to express their wants and ideas. Similar to this, speech-activated gadgets can help people with dementia do things by using voice commands, such sending messages or making phone calls.

In addition to these assistive tools, technology has made it easier to provide a variety of complementary and alternative forms of self-care for people with dementia. These methods include apps and websites that provide music therapy, tailored breathing exercises, and sensory stimulation. These self-help methods have the power to reduce stress, support emotional health, and improve cognitive performance in general.

To conclude, the use of technology in the management of dementia is extensive and constantly changing. The quality of life for people with dementia may be improved by assistive technologies, virtual reality therapies, remote monitoring systems, and different self-help methods. These interventions may also improve cognitive function and communication. I urge people with dementia and their carers to take use of the opportunities that technology offers as a medical professional and health and wellness coach. People can benefit from increased independence, better overall results, and enhanced well-being by implementing these developments into their dementia care plan.

Ethical Considerations in Dementia Care

One of the cornerstones of healthcare is informed consent, which has even more significance when discussing dementia treatment. Cognitive decline is a common symptom of dementia, and it can affect a person's ability to make decisions regarding their own care. Making sure that people with dementia are given the opportunity to participate in decision-making to the best of their abilities is vital as a healthcare provider.

Using a supported decision-making model is one way to help dementia care providers provide informed consent. Understanding the person's values, interests, and aspirations entails close collaboration with both the person receiving care and their carers. To obtain a thorough grasp of the person's abilities and preferences, it could also entail consulting with other medical specialists, such as psychologists or social workers.

In the context of dementia care, autonomy is still another crucial ethical factor. Like everyone else, people with dementia need to have the freedom to make decisions on their own life to the extent that they are capable of doing so. However, the person's capacity for autonomy may be weakened as the illness worsens. Hence, it is imperative for healthcare practitioners and caregivers to achieve equilibrium between upholding the person's liberty and guaranteeing their security and welfare.

Participating in joint decision-making is one approach to preserve autonomy in dementia care. Even if the dementia patient's ability to make decisions is impaired, this entails actively including them in conversations regarding their care. To assist the individual with understanding their alternatives and the effects of their decisions, methods like visual aids or simplified language may be used. As much autonomy over one's own life as feasible is the aim, together with the support and direction required to guarantee one's wellbeing.

One of the most difficult ethical issues in dementia care is arguably making decisions about end-of-life care. People may eventually lose the ability to communicate their desires for their own end-of-life care as the illness worsens. It is crucial under these circumstances that advance care planning and the individual's values and preferences are discussed by medical experts, caregivers, and family members.

Creating an advance care plan as soon as the disease progresses is one method for handling end-of-life decisions in dementia care. The process entails conversing and recording the individual's desires for their medical care, preferred method of resuscitation, and further end-of-life choices. As the patient's health evolves, the plan should be evaluated on a frequent basis and updated. Healthcare providers and caregivers can guarantee that an individual's wishes are recognised and honoured even in cases when they are unable to articulate them by initiating these discussions at an early stage.

It can be difficult and emotionally taxing to navigate moral conundrums in dementia care. It demands that everyone concerned approach it with compassion and collaboration. It is imperative for healthcare practitioners to acquire the requisite competencies and expertise to adeptly handle ethical dilemmas. This could entail continual learning and instruction in subjects like advanced care planning, communication techniques, and moral decision-making.

In maintaining ethical standards in dementia care, caregivers are equally essential. In order to help students comprehend the ethical dilemmas they can face and come up with solutions, they ought to receive assistance and tools. It is also important to encourage caregivers to get help from medical professionals, support groups, or other caregivers who have experienced similar moral conundrums. This support can ensure the dignity and well-being of the dementia patient while also assisting caregivers in navigating the challenges of dementia care.

Being actively involved in our own care is crucial for those of us living with dementia. We can still participate in the decision-making process even though the illness may impair our cognitive capacities. Informing our caregivers and healthcare providers about our beliefs, preferences, and aspirations is crucial. We can make sure that our autonomy is respected and that our care is in line with our preferences by doing this.

In conclusion, ethical issues are crucial when providing care for dementia patients. The well-being and dignity of people with dementia are greatly dependent on informed consent, autonomy, and end-of-life decision-making. In order to resolve the difficult moral conundrums that may come up, healthcare providers, carers, and dementia patients should collaborate. We may respect the values and choices of people with dementia while still guaranteeing their safety and well-being by using a person-centered approach and participating in shared decision-making.

Advocacy and Awareness

In addition to affecting people and their families, dementia has a significant influence on society as a whole. Raising awareness about the crippling consequences of dementia and advocating for individuals living with it becomes imperative as society struggles with the condition's increasing prevalence. In addition to discussing the societal effects of dementia, efforts to reduce stigma, and projects to create dementia-friendly communities, this subchapter highlights the value of advocacy.

Addressing the difficulties experienced by people with dementia requires advocacy, which is the act of speaking up and supporting a cause. As a physician and health and wellness coach, I have seen firsthand how advocacy can enhance patients' lives. Positive changes in their life and our communities can be facilitated by us standing out for their needs and rights.

Reducing the stigma associated with dementia is one of the most important goals of dementia advocacy. Unfortunately, misconceptions and unfavourable preconceptions about dementia are common. As a result, those suffering from dementia may encounter prejudice, social exclusion, and a lack of assistance. We can dispel these myths and advance a society that is more accepting and caring by increasing knowledge and understanding about dementia.

Various groups and projects have been working relentlessly to improve awareness and understanding in order to overcome the stigma attached to dementia. These initiatives seek to dispel myths and increase compassion for people who are impacted by the illness. We can personalise the experience of having dementia by sharing the narratives of those who have the disease and their families, busting stereotypes and promoting conversation.

Additionally, these initiatives seek to inform and involve policymakers, the general public, and healthcare professionals in the needs of people with dementia. We can guarantee that people have the knowledge necessary to effectively help persons who are living with dementia by ensuring that they are given correct and current information.

Another crucial component of activism is developing communities that are dementia-friendly. A community that welcomes and supports people with dementia and allows them to live and contribute fully is said to be dementia-friendly. These communities provide surroundings and services that enhance the independence and quality of life of individuals with dementia, with a focus on meeting their needs and upholding their dignity.

Communities that are dementia-friendly collaborate across multiple sectors, such as healthcare, transportation, and local businesses, to establish welcoming and encouraging settings. For instance, banks and retail establishments might train their employees to recognise and support people with dementia, and transportation providers might make extra accommodations to meet their needs.

These programmes enhance the general well-being of the community in addition to helping those who are suffering from dementia. Everyone gains when we provide inclusive environments and services that promote social cohesiveness and a sense of belonging. Dementia-friendly societies are essentially the result of a concerted effort to place a high value on understanding, empathy, and compassion.

Advocacy and awareness necessitate cooperative action on a larger scale and are not exclusive to particular initiatives or organisations. Together, communities, governments, and healthcare organisations must develop long-lasting policies and initiatives that assist dementia patients and their families.

I have had the honour of working with numerous organisations and stakeholders as a health and wellness coach to raise awareness of dementia and push for improved support systems. We can make sure that the needs of people with dementia are sufficiently met by interacting with legislators and medical professionals.

In summary, comprehensive dementia management necessitates advocacy and dementia awareness-raising. We can build a society that empowers and supports people with dementia and their families by lessening the stigma associated with the condition and fostering understanding. Initiatives to build dementia-friendly communities also improve the lives of those who are impacted by the illness by promoting social cohesiveness and inclusivity.

As we progress in our quest to become experts in managing dementia, we must acknowledge the transformative potential of advocacy and awareness. Through our collective efforts, we can raise awareness in our communities and actively engage in advocacy activities to build a more compassionate and caring society for people living with dementia. Let's take on the duty of being change agents and advocates and collaborate to create a future in which people with dementia are respected, understood, and given the most compassionate care possible.

Empowering Individuals With Dementia

A difficult and crippling illness, dementia affects millions of individuals globally. I have personally seen the devastation it can do to people and their families as a medical practitioner and health and wellness coach. But I also think there's hope and that people with dementia can live happy, meaningful lives.

It is imperative that we change our attention from the dementia itself to the person who is living with it in order to empower those who have dementia. The concept of person-centered care guarantees that the needs, preferences, and goals of the individual are at the core of their treatment. It respects individual autonomy while accounting for their distinct experiences, values, and beliefs. We can design a care plan that genuinely fits their requirements and supports them in preserving their sense of self if we recognise and value their uniqueness.

One of the most important aspects of empowering people with dementia is to promote their autonomy. Giving children options and, to the degree that they are capable of doing so, including them in decision-making are part of it. This might be as straightforward as giving them the freedom to decide what to eat and wear, or it can be more intricate like include them in conversations about their options for care and treatment. We encourage their freedom and help them feel appreciated and respected by allowing them to make decisions.

Building a feeling of identity and purpose in people with dementia is another essential component of their empowerment. People suffering with dementia frequently lose their memory and cognitive abilities, which causes them to feel lost, confused, and frustrated. We can, however, assist them in preserving a feeling of identity and purpose by assisting them in locating hobbies and pursuits that they can still partake in and enjoy. This can be achieved by taking part in hobbies, seeking creative outlets, or doing things that are consistent with their interests and values. We can assist them in finding happiness and fulfilment in their lives by concentrating on what they still have instead of what they have lost.

Studies have indicated that providing person-centered care, encouraging self-sufficiency, and cultivating a feeling of meaning and self might provide noteworthy benefits for those suffering with dementia. According to a study by Pia Kontos and colleagues, the emotional health, level of autonomy, and quality of life of people with dementia improved when they got person-centered care. In a different study, Phyllis Braak and associates discovered that people felt more empowered and were happier with their treatment when they were allowed to participate in decision-making.

Many tactics and approaches can be used to provide person-centered care, encourage autonomy, and cultivate a sense of purpose and identity. Including people who have dementia in the formulation of their care plan is one such strategy. This can be achieved by holding frequent meetings and conversations in which their wants, preferences, and goals are taken into account and included in the care plan. We can make sure that their opinion is heard and that their care is unique by proactively including them in the decision-making process.

Offering meaningful activities and opportunities for involvement to people suffering from dementia is another tactic. This may be accomplished through interventions and structured programmes that highlight their skills and passions. For instance, it has been demonstrated that recollection therapy, music therapy, and art therapy are beneficial in improving well-being and giving dementia patients a feeling of purpose. People can interact with others, find a creative outlet, and feel a feeling of success through these activities.

Apart from these tactics, it is crucial to offer assistance and instruction to both dementia patients and their carers. Many people who suffer from dementia may experience difficulties maintaining their sense of self and a sensation of being powerless over their life. We can help them comprehend and navigate their path with greater confidence and resilience by educating them about their disease and arming them with knowledge. Additionally, caregivers are essential in helping people with dementia feel more empowered. We can empower them to foster an environment that is both powerful and helpful for their loved ones by giving them the resources, tools, and assistance they require.

Giving people with dementia more agency is a complex and continuous process. It necessitates a change in how we provide care and a dedication to treating people with kindness, decency, and respect. We can support individuals in maintaining their sense of self and leading meaningful lives even in the face of dementia by emphasising their individuality, encouraging autonomy, and cultivating a sense of purpose and identity.

To sum up, empowering people with dementia involves appreciating their uniqueness, encouraging their independence, and cultivating a feeling of identity and purpose. Through the implementation of person-centered care, decision-making involvement, and meaningful engagement opportunities, we may assist persons in preserving their sense of self and quality of life. Empowerment necessitates a comprehensive strategy that includes psychological, social, and emotional support in addition to medical measures. Together, we can enable those who are suffering from dementia to live fulfilling lives and with dignity.

The Role of Caregivers and Support Networks

I have direct experience with the effects that carers and support systems can have on people with dementia as a medical practitioner and health and wellness coach. Caretakers have an obligation to provide these people with compassionate and understanding round-the-clock care and support, as these people frequently need it.

Because caregivers are in charge of organising and carrying out the different facets of care, they are essential to the treatment of dementia. This include duties including managing medications, keeping the environment safe, helping with daily living activities, and offering emotional support. Providing care for an individual with dementia can be a daunting and taxing task, but with the correct support system in place, caregivers can successfully navigate these difficulties.

Collaboration is one of the most important elements of effective dementia care. In order to create a thorough care plan that takes into account the specific needs of the person with dementia, caregivers must collaborate with medical specialists such as doctors, nurses, psychologists, and therapists. This kind of cooperation makes it possible to provide care that is holistic in nature, considering every facet of the patient's health and welfare. Together, caregivers and medical experts can make sure that the dementia patient gets the greatest support and care available.

The management of dementia also requires effective communication. To make sure the patient's requirements are recognised and satisfied, effective communication between caregivers and medical experts is crucial. In order for healthcare providers to offer direction and support, caregivers must be able to properly convey any changes or concerns to them. On the other hand, in order to enable caregivers to deliver the best care possible, healthcare providers need to be able to convey crucial information and suggestions to them.

Furthermore, communication within the support system is essential. In order to help with caregiving responsibilities, caregivers frequently rely on the assistance of friends, family, and community groups. The wellbeing of the person with dementia and the caregiver is greatly dependent upon this support system. Ensuring that all members of the support network are in sync and collaborating towards the shared objective of delivering optimal care and support can be achieved through consistent communication and updates.

Having access to resources is also crucial for managing dementia. The resources offered to caregivers are numerous and include financial aid, educational initiatives, support groups, and respite care services. By giving caregivers the information and resources they need to meet the challenges of dementia caregiving, these materials can offer them priceless support and direction. Utilizing these services is crucial for caregivers since they can lower costs related to caregiving and significantly improve the quality of care given.

From my own experience, I have seen the transformation that can happen when support networks and caregivers work together to offer the best possible care and assistance. I have witnessed caregivers go above and beyond to meet the requirements of their loved ones who are suffering from dementia; they persistently fight for their comfort and well-being. I have also seen firsthand the beneficial effects that a robust support system can have on a caregiver's personal health by offering them the psychological and practical assistance they require to perform their caring responsibilities with effectiveness.

It is imperative to recognise the obstacles that caregivers encounter. Providing care for an individual suffering from dementia can be psychologically, emotionally, and physically taxing. Caregivers may find it difficult to get understanding and support from people who have not personally encountered dementia, thus it can frequently feel like a lonely and solitary journey. Formal or informal support networks are therefore crucial. They offer a forum for caregivers to talk about their experiences, ask for guidance, and feel better knowing they're not alone.

In conclusion, networks of support and caregivers are essential to the management of dementia. To provide the best possible care and assistance for people with dementia, caregivers, medical professionals, and support systems must work together. Caregivers can deal with the difficulties of providing dementia care with compassion and skill by cooperating, speaking clearly, and making use of the resources that are available. Having the correct support system in place can also give caregivers comfort, self-determination, and the fortitude to succeed in their caring position.

Future Directions in Dementia Research and Care

I am always investigating new breakthroughs and improvements in the field of dementia research and care as a medical doctor and health and wellness coach. Recent years have seen significant advancements in our understanding of dementia, and with every new finding, we get one step closer to developing more potent therapies and management plans for this crippling illness.

The emphasis on early identification and intervention is one new development in the field of dementia research. We now understand that years or even decades before symptoms appear, the brain alterations linked to dementia can start. We can potentially intervene and slow down the disease's progression if we can recognise the early indicators of cognitive loss. Researchers have recently begun looking into the use of biomarkers—specific proteins or genetic markers, for example—that can detect dementia even in the absence of symptoms. Imaging methods like PET scans or spinal fluid analysis can identify these indicators. This groundbreaking work has implications for targeted therapy and early diagnosis.

An intriguing study topic is the investigation of lifestyle adjustments for the management and prevention of dementia. It is well known that a number of lifestyle choices, including those related to nutrition, exercise, social interaction, and cognitive stimulation, can significantly lower the risk of dementia. The difficulty, nevertheless, is in comprehending how these variables precisely function and how to best utilise them. The current focus of study is on pinpointing the precise food habits, workout routines, and cognitive training plans that will improve brain health the greatest. These results will aid in the development of more focused advice for those who are susceptible to dementia as well as practical tactics for those who are now afflicted.

New pharmacological remedies are being researched and evaluated in the field of treatment. Memantine and other cholinesterase inhibitors are examples of traditional medication therapy for dementia that have somewhat relieved symptoms but do not stop the disease's progression. Currently, scientists are trying to create drugs that specifically target the brain tangles and amyloid plaque buildup that are the fundamental causes of dementia. These cutting-edge medications seek to either prevent the development of these aberrant protein deposits or improve the brain's capacity to eliminate them. Even though these medications are still in the experimental phase, the initial outcomes are positive and suggest that more potent therapy alternatives may be available in the future.

The creation of non-pharmacological dementia treatments is another field of study that has a lot of promise. Researchers and medical experts now acknowledge the value of a multifaceted approach to dementia care as dementia research has advanced. This method incorporates a number of holistic therapies and interventions in addition to medication. Reminiscence therapy, art therapy, music therapy, and aromatherapy, for instance, have demonstrated encouraging outcomes in enhancing the quality of life and lowering behavioural symptoms in dementia patients. Opportunities for self-expression, sensory stimulation, and emotional connection are offered by these non-pharmacological therapies, all of which are critical for preserving cognitive function and general wellbeing. Subsequent investigations will centre on improving and verifying existing therapies, in addition to investigating novel strategies that may augment the quality of life for both dementia patients and their carers.

However, there are a number of issues and barriers in the field of dementia care and research that need to be resolved. The requirement for interdisciplinary collaboration and the integration of information and expertise from other fields—psychology, neurobiology, geriatrics, neurology, and psychology, among others—is one of the major hurdles.

Given the complexity of dementia and its varied aetiology, treating it calls for an all-encompassing strategy. Bringing together specialists from many fields can help us develop more effective preventive, diagnosis, and management measures as well as a more nuanced understanding of the problem.

The involvement and recruitment of a variety of demographics in dementia research is another difficulty. In the past, the majority of the study in this sector has been done on middle-aged or older, white people. Our capacity to completely comprehend the effects of dementia in various communities and to recognise any variations in risk factors, symptoms, and treatment response is hampered by this inadequate representation. In an attempt to surmount this obstacle, scientists are currently endeavouring to incorporate participants from a range of ethnic, cultural, and socioeconomic backgrounds into their investigations. This will assist eliminate health inequities and guarantee fair access to care for all dementia patients, in addition to enhancing the generalizability of study findings.

Despite these obstacles, the field of dementia research and care is full of promise and hope. We are getting closer to a time where dementia is not a death sentence but rather an illness that can be properly treated and even prevented with every new finding and advancement. I'm dedicated to remaining on the cutting edge of these developments as a medical professional and health and wellness coach so that I can give my patients the finest care possible.

In conclusion, there are a lot of opportunities for dementia research and care in the future. There is a growing realisation that dementia necessitates a comprehensive and multifaceted strategy, ranging from early identification and intervention to lifestyle adjustments, innovative drug therapy, and non-pharmacological approaches. It is necessary to overcome obstacles like inclusiveness of varied communities and interdisciplinary collaboration. Nonetheless, there is no denying the advancements being made, which offers hope to the millions of people suffering with dementia and their loved ones. As long as we keep going, I have faith that we will eventually become experts at managing dementia and be able to give people the care, support, and quality of life they need.

Milton Keynes UK
Ingram Content Group UK Ltd.
UKHW020246221123
432980UK00016B/956